Susie Miller founded The FRESH Network, an international help and support organisation based in the UK that co-ordinates information about intuitive raw food diets. For many years she studied human behaviour and psychology, particularly in relation to self-empowerment, and has taught courses in relaxation, meditation and intuitive eating. Currently involved in exploring childhood circumstances which influence the behavioural, emotional and physical health in the emerging adult, Susie now works closely with other families to encourage holistic, self-directed well-being for children and their carers. She lives in rural Devon with her three children.

Karen Knowler worked in the fields of natural health and spiritual development before taking over from Susie Miller as the co-ordinator of The FRESH Network in 1998. Through her writing, speaking and work with the media, Karen teaches others how to discover and explore their own vibrant health potential. Karen lives in Ely, Cambridgeshire.

feel-good food

A GUIDE TO INTUITIVE EATING

Susie Miller & Karen Knowler

*To his Royal Tea-ness
with love &
fruity things!
Karen x*

The information, suggestions and observations included in this book are based on the authors' own experiences. They are offered for educational purposes only and are not intended to be prescriptive.

Therefore, the authors and publishers cannot be held liable for any ill-effects arising from use of any of the suggestions, procedures or recipes contained herein.

This book is not intended as a substitute for professional advice. Anyone who has a medical condition, or is concerned about their health, is advised to consult with a qualified practitioner before making changes to their diet.

First published by The Women's Press Ltd, 2000
A member of the Namara Group
34 Great Sutton Street, London EC1V 0LQ

British Library Cataloguing-in-Publication Data
A catalogue record for this book is available from the British Library.

ISBN 0 7043 4546 3

Typeset by FiSH Books, London
Printed and bound by Cox & Wyman, Reading, Berkshire

Contents

1: Introduction – What is Intuitive Eating?   1
2: The Inside Story   28
3: Contacting our Own Inner Wisdom   66
4: Making Changes and What to Expect   95
5: Living in the Real World   120
6: Intuitive Children   137
7: A Taste of Living Foods   158

Appendix   216
Notes   217
Recommended Reading   220
Useful Contacts   222
Index   239

1 Introduction – What is Intuitive Eating?

The chaos without

Are you confused about what you should be eating? What's healthy, what's economical – and how about what tastes good? We are living in a world where food advice proliferates – whether it be from books, television programmes, newspaper and magazine articles and even internet sites. Each one seems to have its own opinion about what diet is best for us – it's hard to know just who to believe.

As well as the media affecting our decisions, the high profile of food in the world around us also has its part to play, with restaurants, fast food outlets and convenience foods all becoming more numerous and diverse. Yet, as the range of foods available to us has gone up – which, on the face of it is wonderful – their nutritional properties have subsequently gone way down. For example, with intensive farming and the large-scale use of chemical fertilisers and pesticides since World War II, the vitamin and mineral content of our fruits and vegetables has become considerably less than it was, which is one of the many reasons why people comment that food doesn't taste like it used to.[1] Thankfully we find ourselves at a time when overall awareness of health issues is at an all-time high and, as a result of many well-publicised health scares during the past few years, millions of people the world over have begun to question exactly what they are eating.

Of course, this explosion of information, recipes and advice would be wonderful if it was consistent but new ideas, theories and products are emerging all the time. So who should we ask for reliable information about what we should be eating?

Are you fed up with letting food rule your thoughts, your body – your life? Of constantly looking to outside sources for information? Are you sick and tired of feeling sick and tired? So many of us suffer to some degree with health concerns, whether this be the annual cold or flu, weight problems, lingering headaches or something more serious. Surely we're designed to feel much better than this, to have more energy and not be weighed down with niggling problems on a regular day-to-day basis?

This book offers you the opportunity to find solutions to these dilemmas for yourself. Not only does it present food from a different perspective but it also sets the scene for you to discover the most enjoyable and fulfilling way to eat – for you.

The chaos within

Just as we are unable to think straight or do our job properly in an office littered with papers, it is the same inside our bodies. Over time the body clogs up with various debris, taken in through our food and environment and we gradually lose touch with our senses. Because our body works so hard to keep its system working healthily and efficiently, deterioration appears to happen very slowly, so it is often not until the eleventh hour that the debris on the inside manifests itself as illness or disease on the outside. It is only when something is seriously wrong that we wish we'd taken action sooner. Sadly we tend to assume that getting older means getting sicker, as suffering from chronic ailments is almost regarded as a normal state of being for the elderly. Whether we are ill or not, however, it does appear that most people actually do feel disconnected from their bodies – their inner connection has faded to almost nothing; their body seems to have a life of its own.

Perhaps one of the most common examples of these powerless situations lies with the millions of people who battle daily with their weight. So many feel they weigh too much and this often ends in a love/hate relationship with food that only leads to yet more anxiety and results in further weight gain. The solution, which thankfully the majority of health professionals are now prescribing, is to avoid the temporary dieting programmes and quick fixes, and instead focus *permanently* on changing our eating habits and lifestyle.

But in reality, while the idea of improving our lifestyle may sound attractive, there can be very real obstacles in the way. For instance, are we really expected to genuinely stop wanting chocolate or chips or ignore very real cravings for other fatty or sugary foods? This is fundamentally where 'healthy eating' programmes fall down: for the most part, they appeal to the individual's intellectual understanding together with their will-power to get them to make changes. As you may already know from experience, this is much easier said than done.

For the majority of people, willpower and good intentions can be very short lived, because they take away much of the pleasure that eating can and ought to be. When we are used to enjoying a free reign with food and then suddenly are having to think about how many calories we are consuming and whether we're getting enough nutrients, it can soon begin to seem too much like hard work. If we're not eating the foods we really want to be eating, it's very likely we'll throw up our arms in despair and say 'That's it!' and go and buy the first 'unhealthy' food we can lay our hands on! Indeed it soon becomes apparent that there is actually much more to the whole scenario than simply mind-over-matter – otherwise it would be a breeze.

So how do we get round this? How can we free ourselves from the seemingly never-ending cycle of diet/binge, or more commonly, healthy food/junk food?

The answer is simple – we need to get back in touch with our natural instincts, to follow our intuition. If you are to feel truly happy and confident about the lifestyle choices you are making – not just mentally, or physically, or emotionally, or even ethically – it is vital that you rediscover the natural inner wisdom you were born with and learn how to use it. You are, after all, much more than just a mind and body – you have feelings and cravings and habits, and your own particular list of dietary requirements that need to be satisfied. You need something that is flexible, ever-changing as you change, something that works for you. This holistic approach, one that satisfies every part of you, is the only recipe for long-term success.

This book therefore details a 'whole person' plan that will enable you to access your holistic wisdom. By following your own intuitive guidance as it reawakens, you will eventually begin to make better choices for yourself, leading to not just greater levels of well-being, but also to more self-confidence and higher self-esteem.

Intuitive eating

Intuition is the final (sometimes unconscious) result of responding to a whole host of inner and outer messages which lead us forward in a positive direction. This approach to eating is essentially about getting back in touch with your body, assisting it from the outside by changing your diet and lifestyle, and listening to it from the inside to know which step to take next. This can lead to the exciting realisation that we can be our own gurus after all.

Eating intuitively is nothing new; it is after all something our earliest ancestors did – they got hungry, they searched for food and they ate. End of story, until the next time. Switch to modern day life and the picture is completely different: fast food available on demand 24 hours a day, obsessive behaviours and addictions, degenerative diseases, low energy levels and ill health are now very much the accepted norm. How often do we eat from genuine hunger, and not just for entertainment, to relieve boredom, for emotional reasons or even as a way of unwinding?

Intuitive eating is essentially about learning to listen to the body again, to read its signals for food and then translating these needs into appropriate food choices and behaviours. However, in order to get back in touch with these intuitive feelings you will need to follow some basic guidelines at first. But after that it's completely up to you – you really can eat what you like!

Therefore in the chapters that follow we detail this initial 'awakening' plan and give you the important tools you'll need along the way.

So – forget will-power, forget guilty eating, learn how to value your choices more now whatever you are eating, so that in time you can very gradually change and automatically make the healthiest choices – not because you've been told to or because you feel you should, but because you genuinely want to.

What foods help us to discover our intuition?

One concept that all health 'experts' seem to agree on is: the simpler the food the better – ie the less processing that is done to fresh raw produce, the more goodness it will retain. What most people don't realise, however, is that some food processes – especially processing with heat – not only reduces the food's nutritional value, but can also change its molecular structure to such a degree that the body is unable to recognise and treat the meal as an optimum fuel.

It has been estimated that humans have been on this planet for 2.5 million years and yet before the discovery of fire they survived perfectly adequately without cooking a thing! As the anatomy of our digestive organs and our process of assimilation have barely changed over this entire history, one cannot say that we have physiologically adapted to cooked foods. And so, as our bodies were designed to work with simple raw foods, no wonder the signals get confused when molecularly altered foods (ie cooked) go down the gullet!

The proof is not just in the theory, but in the practice. When a simpler, more natural diet has been followed for a while it's astonishing how clear nutritional signals become. Addictive cravings, such as for chocolate or wheat products can disappear altogether – without any will-power whatsoever! This is incredible if you consider that Susie used to be a serious chocoholic, and heaven for her was several bowls of ice-cream covered in golden syrup, while Karen once couldn't conceive of a day being complete without a burger and chips.

In the pages that follow we investigate how, by gradually increasing the amount of simple and raw foods in your diet, eating can once again become the luscious pleasure it was meant to be. Out the door go guilty feelings, confusions about what is healthy, and food intolerances as well as other possible diet-related illnesses. In come revitalised taste buds and food that looks and tastes delicious and feels divine on the inside too.

Once your intuition is back working for you, then as everyone is so unique, it will show you what is best to eat – raw or otherwise – and your own rules can then apply.

What can this book do for you?

This book could radically change your life. This may sound like an overstatement, but you could well find that by learning to listen to and follow your intuition, your energy levels soar, your confidence and self-esteem blossom, your health improves in so many ways and all because you are following you, trusting your own wisdom, becoming a more empowered and fulfilled person!

To introduce this process of awakening the intuition, in 'The Inside Story' (Chapter 2), we look at how the human body works – which food-fuels are the most efficient and beneficial to us, and why. We illustrate how the whole system is adversely affected by using less optimum foods – leading to a warp in our very own instinctive skills which in turn leads to self-destructive habits.

In Chapter 3, 'Contacting our Own Inner Wisdom', we show you how, by using simple skills, you can start to listen more intently to the whole range of inner and outer messages that constantly surround you, greatly influencing your food choices. By combining the biological knowledge with your own thoughts, feelings and experiences you can set the wheels in motion to become your own nutritional expert. As part of this holistic package we take into account not just the food itself but your social and emotional needs, your cravings, economic constraints, habits and any other outside influences that may affect you.

We also show the importance of 'backsliding' and how this is a very useful tool for the whole process. Forget guilt trips over eating 'inappropriately' – times like these provide an invaluable way of understanding yourself better.

'Making Changes and What to Expect' (Chapter 4), explains what you can anticipate as you begin to eat more appropriate foods. By using the awakening plan, you'll start to find that your body regains more energy and you'll begin to experience more vibrant health. In this chapter you will learn what the healing and strengthening signs are – both physically and emotionally – and how you can help yourself during these processes. This is where it gets really exciting as you start to see some incredible changes in yourself!

Chapter 5, 'Living in the Real World', shows you how to thrive with your new eating patterns in your everyday life – for instance, what to say to your family, friends and colleagues who want to know what you're eating and why. We also look at eating out and other social occasions such as dinner parties, weddings and holiday times.

For those with children, 'Intuitive Children' (Chapter 6), explores the complex issues of how to encourage children to use their own intuition and to choose healthy foods enthusiastically. And for those contemplating having a baby, we look at how to give them the best start in life while allowing them the freedom eventually to choose their own foods too.

Western cultures are awash with recipe books and perhaps this is a reflection of the ever-growing dissatisfaction many people have from the foods they eat, often putting a great deal of energy into looking for the 'new' experience that will make foods more palatable and exciting. The resulting meals tend to become progressively highly flavoured, or spicier. However, as tasty as these meals may seem, over time they actually contribute to making the person's taste-buds become more de-sensitised, which continues this dissatisfaction spiral. But with time, as you follow this 'awakening plan' and your body cleanses, gets healthier, more vibrant and more sensitive, your taste buds will gradually come alive again. Consequently the simplest of foods gain an amazing new attractiveness, and the processed foods just don't taste good anymore. So you're not left feeling stranded, wondering what on earth you're going to eat, in Chapter 7, 'A Taste of Living Foods', we show you how to experiment with the simplest ingredients and how to let your intuition guide you to the foods you want and need. The chances are that you will be amazed at just how many delicious new foods there are to try. We also give you some simple – and, for your early days, more complex – strongly flavoured raw recipes to try.

This book comes from a deep inner passion we both share of wanting to help others to help themselves. We are not traditional nutritional experts but have – through exploring health, diet and self-esteem –

discovered ways to empower people to become their own true experts.

The stories of our own dietary lives which follow will enable you to see how, independently, we both found our own intuitive direction. Since those early days we have researched the subject in great depth and have found that intuitive eating really is a way of setting people free. Intuitive eaters become their own authority, using the knowledge and wisdom of others as and when necessary, but equally being able to judge for themselves what is best for their own completely unique wants, needs and circumstances.

Susie's story

Born in 1963, I enjoyed a very traditional, suburban childhood in south-east England with three brothers and working parents.

My mother did not show any great interest in nutrition, but trusted the basics she had gleaned from her own upbringing and the health information on offer at the time. We had quite a range of foods including a few convenience foods like fish fingers, processed cheeses and packaged meat slices. In those early years my mother didn't seem to really enjoy the food preparation process, so our fare was simple and easy – quite understandable considering she was bringing up four children and working too!

At the age of fifteen, however, I decided to switch to

an ethically based vegetarian diet. This was quite a shock to my mother. In those days information on vegetarianism wasn't easily available, so her main concern was whether I was getting enough protein. It's amazing how this protein thing is so heavily embedded in our culture. If only more people knew just what happens when they eat too much protein, as practised by most people in the Western world (see Chapter 3).

In those days I had high vegan ideals, and yet could not conceive of ever living without cheese and eggs. So I became a lacto-vegetarian and took on most of my own food preparation – something that was very new to me.

Along with my strong ethical views about animal welfare, I think a key factor behind my food changes was my teenage emergence to greater self-reliance. To me, this meant that I needed to have more control over my life and what I ate. I was a very rebellious teenager and didn't like anybody having authority over me. My presence at home and school was challenging to all those I came into contact with: I argued incessantly against rules which affected me that I felt were not necessary. The roots of my self-empowerment grew with dramatic force!

However, along with wanting more control over my life, there was a deep background of very low self-esteem and especially not liking my body shape. With three brothers, I was brought up to be intelligent and an achiever. Physical looks were much less important, but like all teenagers in England I was surrounded by images of pencil-thin models. I relentlessly started the journey to whittle away my plump pubescent structure. My new control over my food, my passionate drive to succeed, along with a deep urge to want to fade away and not to face my emerging sexuality gave me the perfect scenario for self-starvation. And I was very successful at it – faking my meals to my mother and getting a real buzz out of finding out just how little I could eat without conspicuously passing out.

I was very fortunate – my strong streak of stubbornness and hatred of being controlled eventually saved me from hospitalisation and the real health risks of anorexia. My mother did just the right thing for me – she threatened that if I did not eat more she would get me hospitalised and tube fed. Horror of horrors, the thought of someone in a white coat forcibly feeding me was enough to break the spell of self-starvation. So I made a fundamental decision to look after myself constructively, get better informed, eat more, and stay in control. In this way I kept my independence, gained some weight and left home.

But I had learnt a crucial lesson. I had a deep sense that only I knew how best to take care of myself.

I had already started my slow journey in search of more and more keys to unlock the door to the 'healthy me'. I reckoned that if I was healthier, I would be stronger, more able to get what I wanted out of life. This was in stark contrast to the weak, fading-away self I had left behind.

I had to nearly starve myself to death before taking that very first step, but once the move was made, the journey took on its own effortless momentum. Gaining more and more aliveness was definitely very addictive and attractive – the sparkle in my eyes was returning and I felt the world was my oyster. I had so much more energy to pursue my real passions, instead of thinking every second about what I could, or more likely couldn't, eat.

The calorie books got thrown out and at a slow pace, along with a very busy life, I started to find out about various aspects of holistic health and natural living. Food became just one factor of many and had lost its stranglehold on my day-to-day life.

With the passing years I had a family of two children and, as I naturally wanted the absolute best for them, once again I started questioning nutrition. By now I had an inkling of suspicion regarding the powerful influence of food producers on the available nutritional research and the resulting guidelines, so I was not going to take the advice of the standard authorities as impartial. As in so many other situations in those early years, I was following my own feelings on things; trusting my own instinct, and then using intellectual back-up to prove my points.

I started this searching process by letting my diet

become simpler: out went the junk and the convenience foods and in came the organic wholefoods. Tinned and packet foods just didn't taste good any more, and I especially hated any lingering aftertaste. I effortlessly lost the desire for dairy foods and in came whole grains, home-made bread, no salt, no sugar, and especially no monosodium glutamate and other flavour-enhancers. I felt these were just used by food processors to mask the cheap taste of unwholesome ingredients.

Along with the food/health quest came a renewed interest in self-awareness and meditation techniques. I knew that health could not be achieved by nutrition alone. I also found that the voice inside my head was not always right, and I wanted to find a way beyond its power. For surely that was the voice which had, so many years ago, told me to starve myself in order to fade away?

So I allowed myself free rein with food. I just ate what I wanted, when I wanted, and found that increasingly I chose raw foods. I chose foods I enjoyed most and which felt really good in my body, not only while eating but for hours afterwards as well. I loved my food more than I had ever done before, even in my chocolate and ice-cream days, so denial was the last thing on my mind!

My diet was radically changing and yet I did not really notice this until reaching a point when cooked food no longer had any appeal for me. Naturally, some alarm bells rang. What if I was harming myself again, trying to fade away with all this light food? I knew I wasn't, but now was the time to investigate the scientific nutritional facts again for clarity.

It's incredible how a lot of people believe every 'fact' just because they see it in print! I was not naïve enough to trust only one author and I widened my search as I needed more reassurance and in-depth nutritional advice for me and my children. Up to this point I had only been self-experimenting because I wanted to stay very safe with the children's nutrition and only change their eating patterns when I was totally convinced that I had found something better for them.

Gradually, over the next few months, I picked up the vital elements of raw nutrition and was very inspired by what I found. The information was radical but felt so accurate that I was driven to set up an information service for others searching for similar support here in the UK and in the rest of Europe. I was very fortunate to be supported by my husband so that I could devote a lot of my time to researching raw food information around the world, without having to earn my living this way. The resulting 'raw food service' was named The FRESH Network. It operated very cheaply as it could be run from my home and did not have to pay any wages. I could then dive headlong into information-seeking, contacting universities, health centres and individuals worldwide.

So now I was finding the scientific information backup to my initial instinctive food choices and everything seemed to fall into place. I had trusted my feelings and had been led to a very vibrant sense of well-being that I could already feel pulsating through my body. No wonder I wanted to shout about it.

Naturally I wanted to change the eating habits of my husband and children. It is only human to want to provide the very best for one's loved ones. By now I was convinced that raw foods were so much more superior to my family's current cooked foods that I felt surely this had to change if I wanted to give them the very best too.

However, trying to change my family's ways became one of my greatest lessons about the importance of not imposing our belief systems on others. No matter how well intentioned these ideas were, I now see how vital it is to teach self-empowerment to our children and to encourage it in others. The children of today are the adults of tomorrow and need to learn how to become gradually more self-reliant. This is more fully explained in Chapter 6.

I soon saw that my husband and children needed room for manoeuvre. Meals evolved and some simple cooked foods returned. The stringent guidelines disappeared and I spent time encouraging my family to learn to listen to their bodies, to value themselves fully and therefore to start their own process of eating for deep overall pleasure and not just to please their taste buds or fit in with my ideas. I learnt how not to force others to eat my favourite foods and, at the same time, reinforced my own drive to empower and inspire others.

The next step was a very unexpected surprise. Much to my delight I was expecting another child after an eight-year gap so I had an opportunity to explore diet in relation to pregnancy, childbirth and babyhood. Would my intuition take me to different food choices again?

My pregnancy went like a dream. After an initial period of early-morning sickness that I had also had with my previous pregnancies (and which I will expand on later in this book), I enjoyed making elaborate meals of top-quality raw food to make a top-quality baby! I had a natural, very short, medication-free and almost pain-free birth at home. Again I had followed my intuition in the way I wanted to birth my new daughter.

I don't know what my next step will be. I now have three children all with different personalities and needs and it's my challenge to give them – as well as myself – the space to explore themselves and their world.

Karen's story

Until the age of about eighteen, my diet was something I didn't really think about too much. If I did, it was in terms of fat grams and calories because that's what mattered to a curvaceous girl like me. My main considerations were, first, that I shouldn't get any fatter and, second, that I wouldn't have to give up chips! Food was both my enemy and my friend, depending on whether I was looking in the mirror or enjoying a favourite meal.

During my teens I must have put on about 20lb, and very quickly, but I wasn't growing taller – only wider! I didn't like what I saw or how I felt and, being a teenager, image was fast becoming an issue. This was when I reluctantly realised that action was needed – but what?

I was born in England in 1972, an only child to two young parents, both of whom were raised on high-fat and processed diets. It wasn't long before my huge appetite (and searching for nutrients) made itself clearly known and as my mother was not confident about breastfeeding, I was switched to cow's milk after only six weeks.

I now see clearly that as a result of my intolerance to dairy products I spent the first six years of my life experiencing mild eczema and colds that lasted for six weeks at a time. I also never slept for very long and was hyperactive. My mother didn't know what to do with me. Both family and doctors alike cited my long colds and hyperactivity as 'just one of those things', and so we accepted it as such.

Over the years my sinuses became more and more congested. When I had these colds I couldn't breathe properly and it was affecting my sleep, so eventually the doctors decided that the best course of action was to remove my adenoids.

My diet during childhood consisted mainly of meat (all kinds), fish, cheese, butter, white bread, baked beans, chips, crisps, biscuits, ice cream, sweets and chocolate, and by school age I wouldn't touch any vegetables. The only exceptions to this were potatoes (fried), mushrooms (grilled in butter) and sometimes, if I was in a good mood, I could be persuaded to eat a few boiled peas! Overall it was a diet exceptionally high in sugar and processed fatty foods, and I could not be persuaded to experiment with anything even vaguely healthy. I just didn't like the taste of such foods. Vegetables made me feel sick, rice actually made me sick, boiled potatoes tasted bland and of nothingness, water tasted disgusting and I could only drink strong squashes, thick creamy milk shakes or sugar-packed fizzy drinks. My parents despaired of me at times, because I didn't like anything but junk! But why should I change when I felt fine as I was?

In my early teenage years my diet became worse still. In my spare time I began working in my stepfather's grocery and butcher's shop, so meat became an even bigger part of my life. I was still eating no breakfast – maybe the odd bacon sandwich now and again – and my childhood lunchbox had been replaced by the cheap, quick-and-easy plate of chips from the school canteen. Sometimes this was accompanied by a slice of pizza, a hot dog or a burger in a roll, and *always* smothered in ketchup. At break times I would usually have a packet of crisps or a chocolate bar. Once back from school I would call into our shop to buy another bar of chocolate, and sometimes this would be accompanied by a whole pint of full-fat milk – straight from the bottle! My evening meal remained as before – always something with chips, the occasional cheese or ham salad in the summer, but I was still not eating many vegetables.

And so it went on until – boys!

Now at high school, I began to become more and more conscious of the way I looked. Surprisingly, I had not been overweight until puberty – a body can hold itself together quite well while it's young and active – but aged only fifteen, things were definitely taking a turn for the worse. A low-fat diet helped as long as I was following it, but – real life intervened – I got bored, my habits reverted. I didn't like having to go out of my way to find low-fat foods when convenience foods were all around me. Besides, I loved chips and cookies, and I wasn't *that* big. I still cycled to school and played netball regularly; I even swam and played squash occasionally. In fact I was one of the sportiest girls in my year; generally I felt fine.

However, at the age of seventeen it finally hit me that my body was slowly degenerating. I arrived home from a sixth-form exchange trip to America, and found that due to overindulging considerably while there, my weight had reached a rather hefty 140lb, and all on a five-foot four-inch frame. Not only that. My eyes were dull and lifeless, my skin was pale, I felt miserable, frustrated and angry. Why couldn't I control myself? The worst thing of all was that my cellulite – the bane of so many women – wasn't simply on my thighs and bottom (though that was bad enough) but also in my arms, stomach and knees. I hated what I saw, and it was *me*.

With the evidence before my eyes, I could no longer pretend it wasn't happening. It was hard. I wasn't even into my twenties and already my body was on a visibly downward spiral. I had no real idea of how to reverse the momentum. I didn't dare even imagine how I would look in another decade or two. It was time to check out the options more seriously.

Over the next year I reintroduced the low-fat rule into my life. Once more I cut down on the frequency and amount of fried foods I ate – I grilled instead. I stopped having butter on my bread. I followed the magazine tips for switching one food for a healthier lower-fat option, and my shape changed and my weight went down.

Little did I know it then, but that was just the beginning of my investigations. The more I thought about food and its impact on the human body, the more questions I had. Why should people have to battle with their weight at all? Why could some people eat apparent rubbish and still be slim? What exactly do those additives do inside the body? Why are healthy foods healthy? But the question I really wanted to find the answer to was: is it possible to love food and be slim *and* healthy?

The first major change for me was in 1992 when I went to live with my father and stepmother. It was the first time I had ever seen a different example of how other people eat on a regular day-to-day basis. It was a real education. Instead of a white sliced loaf, there was freshly baked wholemeal bread. Instead of bacon there was lean ham; tuna instead of cod in batter; and so on. At last I could actually try a different way of eating.

Considering my passion for burgers and my loathing for vegetables, it did seem rather ironic that I spent four of my teenage years toying with the idea of going vegetarian. It wasn't so much that I didn't enjoy eating meat; I found that my ethical concerns were becoming increasingly important to me and were beginning to override every other consideration. But what could I do? No meat and no veg? What exactly *would* I eat?

In May 1992, only four months after moving in with my father and his family and aged nineteen, I decided I could finally do without meat. By this time my stepmother had proved to me that vegetarian dishes could in fact be extremely delicious! A miracle had happened – I was eating and actually enjoying vegetables! In no time at all I was eating things like muesli, baked potatoes, coleslaw, tuna and rice.

Progress indeed. I was even eating fruit and yogurts for snacks. What really surprised me, however, was the fact that I was genuinely enjoying my new way of eating. It was *really* tasty.

Three months later I was living in London and catering for myself for the first time. It was then that my progress quickened. Due to my own concern and the friendly concern of others, I intended to arm myself with all the knowledge necessary to assure them, and myself, that I was eating a healthy diet. So I read and read until I was soon eating just fruit until lunchtime (to assist with the body's natural elimination cycle) and increasing the amount of more wholesome, natural foods in my diet during my lunchtime and evening meals. I also experimented with the principles of food combining (see Chapter 2).

In fact, the more I experimented the more I learnt that my body would show me what it did and didn't like. When I was eating out I would actually choose a jacket potato and salad over quiche and chips every time … and I wasn't even trying. I didn't need to convince myself of anything, I just ate whatever made sense to me, and without exception found that it really worked. I did feel better! I did feel more alive! I had more energy to do more things and life began to seem full of possibilities. The pale-faced girl of just a year ago was slowly bringing herself back from the dead!

Over the next few months my discoveries came thick

and fast. I read so many books on so many subjects related to diet and health that my intellectual understanding grew and grew. But I was also experimenting with 'power foods' like Spirulina, for example. The first time I tried it (I made a banana smoothie with it) I was almost bouncing off the walls! Talk about high energy! This food thing was taking me to places I had only dreamt of.

Then I was ready for the next step – a trial run of veganism. I knew this would be a bit of a challenge because of social situations and what others might say, but the idea of veganism appealed to me immensely after an experimental period of going without milk. This had led me finally to being congestion-free. I was interested to see how I would get on without cheese, butter, mayonnaise and eggs. I really wasn't eating much of them anyway.

It was at this point that I realised that I would have to add more variety to my menu if I was to be a *healthy* vegan. Thank goodness for Leslie Kenton's work then. Her best-selling book *Raw Energy* changed my life yet again. Not only was there excellent information available on plant foods and the benefits of eating them raw, but even more new foods to try! Instead of my diet seeming to narrow down to nothingness as is the commonly held view of veganism, a whole new vista opened up. I could be vegan *and* eat a different meal every day of the year – I had never heard of such tasty dishes in my whole life. Not only that, but the accompanying claims of vibrant health and regeneration of the body through living foods made perfect sense: I was determined to have some of this!

I didn't know it then, but for me that was to be the major turning-point. Over the next five years I experimented continually with varying amounts of living foods in my diet. Sometimes I would go for days, other times weeks, sometimes even months without eating anything cooked, but all the time being guided by what I came to know as my intuition. I didn't have a clue where I was going at times, but it definitely *felt* right. Of course the books all played their part, but it was *living it* that really taught me fact from fiction.

2 The Inside Story

Although it may seem odd to some, awkward to others and downright outlandish to a few, raw food just makes perfect sense once you start. Who would not wish to have improved energy levels, vibrant health, greater resistance to illness and a profound sense of well-being, whilst reducing the impact of their lifestyle on the environment?
Maxine Tuck, veterinary surgeon and sports athlete, UK

Using your intuition is about following your own feelings and not someone else's rules. For most of us, however, this is a skill that needs to be relearnt. In this chapter we explore the scientific reasoning as to why we recommend using specifically raw foods for this awakening process and why you'll probably find this is what you *want* to eat after your intuition is awakened.

Put simply, raw natural plant foods are the optimum for our physiology and consequently they present the most straightforward pathway to uncovering our ability to eat intuitively.

We begin this chapter with a wide overview of the animal kingdom to see where humans fit in. By outlining the basic differences and similarities in physiology between us and other species, we can start to recognise the multitude of clues that show us which diet we are best suited to and why.

The second section focuses on our bodies as a unit, outlining why things work the way they do and why things go wrong. This leads on to the nitty-gritty of food and nutrition and the vital role that has to play in our overall health and vitality.

By considering the facts discussed in the following pages, we hope that you will begin to feel confident that physiologically, biologically and chemically our bodies are designed to thrive on fresh, ripe, unprocessed organic plant foods. By eating in this way we put ourselves on track for achieving outstanding levels of health – our natural birthright.

The human animal

Most of us do not live what would be considered to be natural lives any more and our lifestyles in general are a far cry from those of our distant ancestors. We live in robust, indoor homes, hiding from the natural elements and surrounded by the trappings of modern living. But have our bodies really adapted and changed physiologically because of our change in environment?

We may think that we have somehow evolved, and to

some extent this is true – we have survived and made it this far. But the truth is that our physiology is practically the same today as it always has been since the emergence of our species, *Homo sapiens*.

Body clues

Fundamentally, we are just an animal species. By comparing our physiology to other animal groups, we can gain many useful clues to the structure of our ideal diet. The following information is adapted from *Psycho-Psysiopathy* by Dr T. De la Torre.[1]

Starting with the face, our eyes point forward, with restricted peripheral vision – try looking round to the side without moving your head and you'll notice that your vision is extremely limited. When observing other animals, we learn that it is the hunters and not the hunted who have forward-pointing eyes. However, carnivorous animals also have stereoscopic vision which enables them to see all around them, so as to hunt down prey at a moment's notice. Humans, like the anthropoids such as apes and monkeys, have forward vision without the stereoscopic range that carnivores have. This suggests a more simple, stable diet of plant foods (which don't run away) and also a more peaceful way of living overall, having no need to hunt or be hunted.

Next, the nose. Our upright stance suggests that we would smell our foods high off the ground or lift food to our noses, rather than sniff around on the ground like carnivores, omnivores and herbivores. Notice, too, how these other animals have their jaw-lines closely shaped around their noses, so they can use their noses at the same time as their mouths in most cases, in order to push the food around. We have our hands for this facility and use our noses only to check for potency, freshness and attractiveness.

Our ears are also set in such a way that suggests we don't need to have sharp hearing in order to secure our next meal. They do not prick up like those of wild animals, instead, like our eyes, they remain alert yet in a relatively peaceful and inactive state.

Of all our facial features our mouth is the most important clue-giver. We chew rather than rip, shred or tear. When we eat our food it is a natural inclination to move our jaw up and down rather than from side to side. Our teeth do not enable us to rip into another animal and tear it limb from limb with relish, or to pull up a mouthful of grass and chew on it, cow-like, for hours upon hours.

Unlike the carnivores and omnivores, our saliva is alkaline, meaning that it is adapted to the digestion of sugars and starches, that is plant foods, and is not at all suited to breaking down animal protein.

Moving down to our stomach, we find yet more evidence: carnivores secrete ten times more hydrochloric acid than us in order to digest flesh, which again suggests that we are not designed to consume flesh.

Finally, the intestines and colon show that our whole digestive and eliminative process is very much geared towards a vegetarian diet. A carnivore's intestinal canal is only 3 times the length of its body whereas we and our closest cousins, the anthropoid apes, have intestinal canals 12 times the length of our body. Likewise the colons of carnivores are short and smooth, designed for prompt evacuation rather than further digestion, whereas ours are long and involved, allowing for the much longer digestion and assimilation of plant foods.

Working on the premise that our body signposts the way towards what foods are right for us, it is helpful to look to those anthropoid apes. Different from us by only 2 per cent of their genes, we can clearly see that, like us, they also spend much of their time upright, they have flat nails and fingers much like ours, and they also feed their young in a very similar way. In fact, the list of similarities goes on and on. These animals are frugivorous – they eat fruit, nuts and leaves. While the idea of being likened to chimpanzees or bonobos genetically may not be especially glamorous, it is feasible to conclude that humans are designed as frugivores too.

Of course, the fact that various members of the human race exist on every kind of diet – from almost totally meat-based through to fruitarian – does mean we can survive on almost anything. Survival is one thing, but are we *thriving* on it? Individually we are doing what we think best, what we enjoy, or what circumstances and climate provide for us, depending on our current life situation. Effectively we are playing a part in what could be viewed as a big experiment, both as individuals and as a whole. Humans are, after all, the only animal to eat such a wide range of foods. Perhaps only now are we truly beginning to understand the long-term consequences of such experimentation.

Unhindering our bodies

The body is a complex, brilliant and finely tuned machine. It should be a great place to live – beautiful, comfortable, light and airy, and designed to last a lifetime with minimal upkeep if treated correctly. Although we are not born with an instruction manual telling us how to look after it, all the knowledge is there already, inbuilt like a program. For instance, if we do something damaging it is very quick to tell us. The most obvious example is when we burn our hand on something, the immediate reaction being to pull away from the offending object. However, when it comes to things we ingest, our senses are rather less acute – not because of anything missing from our programming but quite simply because we have lost touch.

This section outlines the main ways in which you can help your body regain its vitality so that you can restore this connection.

Cleaning the inner debris

Our digestive system is incredible. Digestion actually begins in the mouth as food reacts with our saliva. Upon swallowing, the system takes the food down through the stomach, duodenum, intestines and colon, ingesting the nutrients it is able to and then finally passing any waste matter out through the anus.

The colon (large intestine) is the last port of call for all unused foodstuffs and byproducts of digestion and it is responsible for eliminating toxic wastes that include millions of dead cells and tissues, as well as absorbing nutrients which the small intestine could not. It is here in the colon that many of our health problems begin.

Due to our poor eating and drinking habits, stress, pollution, intake of drugs, inappropriate medications and smoking etc, over time the colon may become impacted with a great deal of uneliminated matter which actually hardens and adheres to its walls.[2] This is sometimes referred to as mucoid plaque and quite probably it afflicts every single person eating a standard Western diet. With each passing year, the coating becomes thicker and more impacted until, in some cases, what was previously a $6^{1}/_{2}$-cm-wide passageway is only a few millimetres wide. As the digestive system is no longer able to adequately utilise the food working its way slowly through, this naturally leads to constipation and malabsorption problems. Such an environment is also an ideal breeding ground for unfriendly bacteria and, ultimately, disease.

A healthy transit time for food to pass through your body from the time of eating to elimination should be 24 hours or less. In the UK the average transit time for women is 70 hours – that is three days – and for men, 60 hours. In fact, the UK is the most constipated nation in the world and has the highest incidence of bowel cancer anywhere, with 20,000 new cases per year. It is estimated that as many as one in every three people sitting in a doctor's surgery is there because of some kind of bowel problem.[3] If a system is clogged up in such a way, there is a great risk of autointoxication. This means that toxins will continue to seep from the colon out to all parts of the body, leading to a wide range of health problems. What it also means is that whatever diet you eat, if your colon isn't clean it is impossible to achieve vibrant health. This is one of the least known aspects of optimum nutrition. In Chapter 4 you can read about two different ways to assess your own particular state of inner cleanliness, and by returning to your natural diet your colon and digestive system will eventually become cleansed.

Cooked food confusions

How does your body react when you ingest a cooked meal? The startling truth is that the body views cooked food as an invader and sets the immune system into action. This condition is known as digestive leucocytosis and refers to the behaviour of the white blood cells within the body when cooked or processed food is eaten. Rather than staying put and doing their usual job of maintaining immunity within all parts of the body, white blood cells immediately detect 'danger' and rush to the intestines, preparing to wage war! Unless you are already eating a largely raw diet, this means that your body's immune system is being compromised every day of your life.

The practice of eating cooked food had become so commonplace that all scientific studies that looked into this phenomenon assumed that digestive leucocytosis was 'normal'. It wasn't until Paul Kouchakoff, a scientist studying at the Institute of Clinical Chemistry in Lausanne in the 1930s, experimented with people eating raw foods that he discovered it didn't happen with them.[4]

Body cycles

As taught by the Eastern philosophy of Ayurveda, the body generally works to three very definite cycles throughout the 24-hour period.[5] These are: appropriation, assimilation and elimination. Although the body can be eating/digesting, using food and cleaning all at the same time to varying degrees, it has been found that from approximately 4 am until noon, the body is cleansing itself – elimination. This is why, for example, people wake up with headaches, crusty eyes, furred tongues and so on – that is the debris coming out. It makes most sense for the body to at least begin its house-cleaning while we are asleep, because it is then that we are not exerting any extra energy and can let nature take its course. During this first eight-hour period, the best foods we can possibly eat are (if hungry, of course) fruits, because they require minimal digestion and are the only ones that have been found not to interfere with the cleansing process. Therefore the ideal scenario is to try to introduce more fruit into your morning routine and slowly cut down on other items.

The second eight-hour cycle, appropriation, is between noon and 8 pm, which is when most of us eat our two main meals of the day. This is the time when the body is most efficient at digesting and dealing with foods. It's also the time when we burn them up the fastest because we are at our most active. At this time – if we're eating according to the dictates of our appetite – we should be refuelling and burning, refuelling and burning, in a fairly steady and comfortable way. Eating when one is truly hungry can take a bit of getting used to, but it is far more enjoyable than eating just because it's lunchtime or we've been offered food and are nervous about refusing.

The third cycle, assimilation, is the time for utilising the food we have consumed during the day. This takes place between 8 pm and 4 am, ie the time we're most likely to be relaxed or least active. Any foods eaten at this time are likely to be digested more slowly, and you may well have experienced waking up with a heavy stomach after eating late at night.

By working in conjunction with these three cycles, you will become much more aware of how real they are.

Food combining

The principles of food combining have become especially well publicised in recent years. It is based on the premise that we shouldn't mix a concentrated source of protein (such as meat or fish) with a carbohydrate (such as bread or potatoes) in the same meal because the two varying food types need different digestive juices to break them down. Therefore the stomach can only work with one type of food at any one time, and if they are mixed, neither gets properly digested – yet another way of contributing to a clogged-up colon.[6] As far as raw-food eating is concerned, you will find, because of the potency of such foods, that the results will be even more marked. For instance, if you eat some sprouted grain or grain crisps with a handful of nuts, you can bet that digestion is going to be very slow indeed, possibly with a dash of flatulence!

As a general rule fruits are best eaten alone because they digest so quickly – if eaten with nuts or grains it is likely to result in fermentation and maybe even discomfort. Fresh leafy greens, herbs and other vegetables are great 'neutral' foods and go well with practically everything.

The system of food combining – remembering which foods should go with which – can be perplexing. However, do remember that all food-combining charts and tables (see Appendix) are only tools, and essentially are based on the inherent wisdom your body *already* possesses. So, instead of putting the process into your brain as a regime of eating, think of it more as a program which is already a part of you. As you learn to listen to your body's signals, you'll learn about food combining firsthand in a way you will never forget.

Body balance

The body is programmed first for survival and second for health, and is continually giving priority to maintaining various key elements such as the pH level (acid/alkali balance), salt concentration, temperature and blood-sugar levels. Homeostasis, which is the balance of all of these and more, is vital for the efficient functioning of the whole system.

Our acid/alkali balance (pH) is measured on a scale of 0 to 14 – 0 is extremely acid, 14 extremely alkaline, and 7 neutral (water is neutral). The human body maintains a blood pH of 7.35 to 7.4, but if it varied by even a small amount (eg down to 7, or up to 7.8), your life would be in grave danger.[7]

Many of the things we Westerners consume on a regular basis are extremely acidic in nature. Each time we ingest one of these our body immediately calls on all its buffers, such as water and minerals, in order to dilute the offending item. This in turn leads to weight gain and water retention due to the body locking any toxic elements away into fat cells and body tissues, so that they're out of harm's way. To redress this acidic imbalance, the body then robs minerals from its own bones, muscles, tissues and ligaments – if this didn't happen, death would be inevitable. This is why blood can appear normal even in those who are seriously ill, because other parts of their body are compensating, all the while becoming very depleted in themselves.[8]

As our body strives to maintain an alkaline state within its systems, our diet therefore should reflect this leaning. Many researchers have suggested that the ideal ratio should be a diet of 80 per cent alkaline-forming foods and 20 per cent acid-forming foods. This aside, a good rule is to focus on making the larger part of your diet alkaline. So which are the most acid-forming? Here follows a list of the biggest offenders: dairy products, refined sugar, white meats (chicken, fish, etc), red meats (beef, pork), coffee and tea, salt, alcohol, drugs and some medications. And which are the best alkaline-producing foods? It's no surprise to find that these are raw fruits and vegetables.

Food facts

Food is the main raw material from which we build our body and, of course, one of the biggest commercial industries in the world.

Our introduction to the world of nutrition usually begins at school, where conventional nutrition charts introduce us to the concept of food groups for the first time. This food pyramid has at its base the grains or 'complex carbohydrates' group, which is presented as the most important area for supplying the body with its energy. This is seconded by a large serving of fruits and vegetables; then follow dairy products, meat and fish, and finally a small amount of processed or sugary foods.

On the face of it, it is easy to think that this is not too far off the mark and, indeed, it is certainly not the worst-case scenario – but it misses so much out. As we will see later, food is of little benefit to us if our body cannot absorb the goodness within it properly.

In this section we take a quick look at the different components within foods and how they interact with each other, and why it is so important that they are kept natural and raw. We then investigate enzymes, a little-known-about, but absolutely vital part of the digestive and health-maintaining process. Enzymes are in fact our lifelong friends and are vital in every bodily function, but we unwittingly kill them off in our food preparations and consequently deplete our own personal enzyme reserves.

This leads us on to the subject of cooking – why is it so damaging? What do we forgo when we heat-treat foods? What about other forms of processing and what do these do to our body?

Nutrition in a pill

Even though we are led to believe otherwise, the subject of nutrition is by no means a complete science. Did you know, for example, that it has been suggested that scientists have discovered only approximately one-tenth of the nutrients they estimate to exist? Only a few decades ago when less than a hundred nutrients had been identified, the estimation was that there would be about another two hundred to find. At the present time, when thousands have been discovered and named, it is estimated that there are at least as many as one hundred thousand![9] As advanced as we may consider ourselves to be in many scientific fields of endeavour, complete nutrition is not yet one of them.

It shouldn't therefore surprise us to learn that there has never been a successful attempt to keep a person – or animal – healthy, or even alive, on a diet of nutritional supplements alone. The other important point about supplements is that most nutrients work symbiotically with at least eight other nutrients[10] – popping a pill of one thing here and another thing there cannot come anywhere near to negotiating the delicate balancing act which wholefoods take care of simply and naturally. In fact it has been shown that some supplements are very poorly absorbed and assimilated by the body, not least because they are usually completely enzyme- and fibre-deficient due to being so highly processed.

This of course doesn't even begin to take into account the fact that what ends up in the bottles of food supplements is what we have cooked or processed out of our foods already!

Cooking effects on the key elements of nutrition

If you want to set the vibrancy of your health on fire, stop setting fire to your food!
Professor Rozalind Gruben, AHSI, RSA,
international health & fitness speaker and consultant, UK

Vitamins

Vitamins are regarded as chemicals, and are absolutely essential for health. Despite scientists' increasing understanding of their chemical structure, what hasn't been discovered is the biochemical role of many of them. To date there are fifteen known vitamins, four of which are fat-soluble and the other nine water-soluble. They act as catalysts and react with proteins, glucose and fats in the body's vital digestive and metabolic processes. Vitamins are altered in structure by exposure to temperatures of over 130°F (approximately 55°C)[11] – bear in mind that a cool oven is set at approximately 225°F! Once damaged by heat they are much more difficult for the body to make use of and are more likely to be eliminated as a toxin, stored as waste within the colon, or deposited elsewhere in the body, often in fat cells. Fruits are the number-one source of vitamins known to humankind.

Minerals

Minerals, also referred to as mineral salts, are most commonly used as building blocks for bones, teeth and cellular tissues. As with vitamins, when overcooked they also become virtually unusable (termed inorganic), and are mostly eliminated or stored away in the tissues.[12] Those who eat a highly acid-forming diet (meats, cooked fats, high protein and so on) are the most likely to have a mineral deficiency owing to the alkalising properties of their own body minerals (such as bone calcium) being used to maintain the correct acid/alkaline balance within the blood and other bodily fluids (as mentioned earlier).

Minerals also transport nutrients to cells and act as electrolytes, carrying electromagnetic currents through the body. As such it is essential that they are consumed through raw plant foods so that their activity remains at vital optimal levels. Generally speaking, vegetables (from the land and sea) are our optimum source of minerals.

Fats

Fats have been given such a bad press in recent years that many of us run off screaming at the mere mention of the word! However, there are good fats as well as bad fats; of course, the so-called bad fats are best avoided, but – and this is a big but – the vast majority of the population, no matter what kind of diet they are eating, are deficient in the fats which really matter. These vital fats are otherwise known as EFAs, that is, essential fatty acids. Our bodies can only gain them through the foods we eat, and currently the typical Western diet, whether it's 'lite', full-fat or anywhere in between, is just not providing enough of them.

There are two main types of fat which most of us are more than familiar with: saturated and unsaturated. Saturated fats are solid fats with a high melting point, and come in the form of animal products such as beef, pork, dairy products and margarines. These fats stick together and form thick droplets or hard plaque within the body, furring up arteries and interfering with many bodily functions. The primary sign of this happening is the onset of high blood pressure; if left unchecked, this can lead to many of the chronic health problems we've all been warned against, not least cardiovascular disease. Refined sugars and starches which aren't used immediately as fuel are also converted to fats and stored within the body.

Unsaturated fats are, generally speaking, the good guys of the fat world, but there are some exceptions. This group is split into two subgroups: mono-unsaturated and polyunsaturated. The polyunsaturated fats are then split into two further subgroups: essential and non-essential fatty acids.

The main difference between saturated and unsaturated fats is that the latter do not stick together in the blood stream and have a much lower melting point (if they are not liquid already). Examples of mono-unsaturated fats are coconut, palm kernel oil, olives, almonds and fresh raw seeds. When eaten in small amounts, these can be very beneficial, keeping the arteries clean and elastic.

Polyunsaturated fats are traditionally the most beneficial all round, though only when eaten in their natural raw state. Hydrogenated oils and fats – that is, fats heated to between 120°C and 210°C – do contain polyunsaturates and so are referred to as such on food labels despite being processed. This is particularly unfortunate as heated fats have become completely different in their chemical make-up and are destructive to the body, if not possibly carcinogenic.[13]

The EFAs are absolutely vital for our all-round well-being – they carry toxins to eliminative organs and transfer oxygen to all the cells, including the brain, resulting in mental vitality. Deficiencies can result in liver and kidney problems, hair loss, miscarriage, retardation, impaired vision and arthritis among other things. Three excellent sources of EFAs are safflower oil, hemp oil and linseed/flax oil, although they can be found in less obvious places such as leafy green vegetables. Good news for those wanting to lose weight – EFAs can increase the metabolic rate, which in turn, increases the body's calorie-burning capacity. So the good fats begin fighting the baddies – and win – by helping to dissolve saturated fatty acids and the harmful cholesterol already stored in the body. The key to obtaining EFAs of optimum quality is that they must be fresh. They must not, therefore, be exposed to light, oxygen or heat – so avoid buying these oils in clear glass bottles (if in doubt ask at your health food store). As usual, the optimum way to get the freshest and purest oils possible is to chew your raw nuts and seeds well or grind them to make your own oils or sprinkles. All nuts, seeds and oils are available from good health food shops or by mail order (see Useful Contacts).

Carbohydrates

The term 'carbohydrate' has commonly been attributed to grain or cereal products – especially bread, pasta, rice and potatoes. However, carbohydrates also refer to all the sugars and starches found within foods, which of course includes fruit and vegetables as well as cereal crops.

Long heralded as 'energy food' and the perfect fuel for athletes due to their rapid absorption into the bloodstream, of all the carbohydrates available to us, fruits, rather than the traditional starchy potato or wheat product, are the best source of fuel for sportspeople. Fruit sugars are far more bio-available to the body, leaving barely a trace of residue and requiring minimal digestion. As digestion takes more energy than any other activity we engage in, it makes sense to minimise our energy expenditure, especially when competing at a high level.

All sugars are rapidly absorbed into the body and, if not burned up, are turned into fats – fats that are difficult to revert back to sugars again. Starches are simply sugar molecules bonded together, thereby making them slightly more complex so that their energy is released more slowly.

The worst kind of carbohydrates for the body are those which have been refined – things such as white breads, pasta, rice and so on. These are practically devoid of vitamins and minerals, thus providing the body with very little nutrition. In fact, due to their lack of fibre and 'completeness', the body is unable to utilise them properly. Consequently their sugars are absorbed much more rapidly into the bloodstream than they would be if they were wholefoods. This triggers the pancreas to secrete insulin in order to rebalance the blood sugar level, which in turn stimulates the conversion of sugars to fats which are then stored in bodily tissues and organs. By continuing this cycle on a regular basis, the risk of triggering hypoglycaemia or diabetes becomes much higher. At best the cravings for sugar, sweets and other less than optimal foods increases, leading to a continuing downward spiral of poor food choices.

Complex carbohydrates are wholefoods such as

potatoes, corn, vegetables, wholegrain rice, and other wholegrains. Being more or less complete foods (depending on their preparation) these are much closer to their original state and therefore easier for the body to deal with. Having a considerably higher vitamin and mineral quotient, as well as containing a large amount of fibre, they are absorbed much more gradually by the body and their release of energy is slower and more balanced. When it comes to the effects of cooking, any carbohydrates which have been heat-treated are absorbed much more quickly than their raw counterparts; again this increases the chances of blood-sugar abnormalities as well as adding to the work needing to be done by the system – especially by the pancreas – in order to maintain body balance.

Proteins

Proteins are made up of amino acids, which in turn are used to maintain body tissues and hormones. There are at least twenty in all, eight of which are termed 'essential' because they must be supplied by the diet. Contrary to popular belief, all fruits and vegetables supply some, many, or all of these essentials. By eating a variety of these foods in their pristine natural state, all of the body's protein needs will be more than adequately met.

For years it was touted that meat was the best source of protein, but science has since found that protein obtained from animal sources is not only unnecessary but potentially harmful.[14] The inside story is that if we were to watch the action of animal protein within the body we would see that with the ingestion of meat, uric acid is introduced to the system as a byproduct. This leads to incredible over-stimulation within the bodily system and calcium is stolen from various parts of the body in order to buffer it and prevent it from doing harm. The calcium then combines with the uric acid and crystals are formed which, if not fully eliminated, can in turn lead to kidney stones, gout and rheumatism.

Cooked proteins – whatever source they come from – are almost completely denatured because their amino acid array has been deranged by heat.[15] They also take the longest of all nutrients to process, thereby putting the most strain on the body.

High protein intake has been shown through numerous studies to lead to premature ageing – a typical example being the Inuit and the African Masai, both of which are very big meat eaters.[16] The average lifespan for such people is between 25 and 45 years. While we in 'developed' countries also consume a high proportion of animal-based proteins, races such as these consume a diet almost entirely consisting of animal products. Note, however, that many Westerners of this age group are also now suffering from heart-related diseases. Evidence is also emerging that high protein consumption can help to cause osteoporosis, as again the body needs to rob from its own bone minerals to counterbalance the acid effect of the excess protein.[17]

Enzymes

Everyone has heard of proteins, carbohydrates, vitamins and minerals, but enzymes? These little powerhouses are rarely mentioned in mainstream health publications, let alone discussed in detail. And yet they are needed for every chemical action and reaction in our body! Briefly, enzymes act as catalysts and are involved in every bodily function – they are commonly regarded as protein molecules carrying an invisible charge, an inner life-force which enables them to affect everything they come into contact with.

Enzymes are found in every organ of our body and can be categorised as one of three different types: the metabolic enzymes for the full functioning of every part within us, the digestive enzymes for food assimilation and those enzymes which are introduced to the body through any raw foods we eat. As our digestive process needs a vast array of enzymes to properly break down our foods, these ideally need to be present in the things we eat. If they are not, the body will use its own reserves. In order to do this it will spend its energy creating extra digestive enzymes instead of keeping the metabolic enzymes in good supply. Children and young people are seemingly able to 'cope' well on an enzyme-depleted diet, but as they get older the true consequences appear: as a depleted metabolic enzyme reserve equates to a less healthy and vital body, it leads to more rapid ageing and susceptibility to illness and disease.

Therefore, if we want to build and maintain vibrant health our focus should be on retaining an optimum level of enzymes while, at the same time, introducing as many new enzymes as possible to our body via our diet. The importance of eating raw natural plant foods here is absolutely key. Raw foods are the only foods that come replete with their own enzymes – they supply between 5 and 40 per cent of the enzymes needed to digest them. By stark contrast, if you eat any cooked foods you contribute the grand sum of 0 per cent to the equation because their enzymes are rendered useless due to the heating process. Not only are they contributing nothing, they are also drawing enormously on the body's reserves, thus leading to a negative balance.

According to extensive research done by Dr Edward Howell (over a period of more than fifty years), once a food is heated to over 48°C/118°F all of the enzymes are completely destroyed. This means that all canned, pasteurised, baked, boiled, roasted, stewed, microwaved, irradiated and fried foods are technically enzyme-empty.[18]

The water of life

As a nation of tea and coffee drinkers, here in the UK we are actively encouraged to drink more water to aid our health. So what do those people drink who follow a high raw diet? The answer is masses of water – perhaps not in a glass or a mug, but directly through the raw produce they eat. It is packed so full of goodness such as assimilable minerals, vitamins and enzymes that it's sometimes called 'living water'.

Because raw foods are extremely high in water that is naturally distilled, they hydrate the body in a gentle, continuous way. In the early days you will probably still want or need to take your liquids separately, in which case there are delicious raw drinks such as fresh juices, nut and seed milks, and smoothies. (See Chapter 7 for more details).

How hot is hot?

We have discussed how the heating process takes away from foods in terms of their nutrient content and, rather worryingly, brings about their complete loss of enzymes. We have also given a few examples of how the body itself views cooked foods biologically. There are ways to process food that aren't as harmful, while continuing to keep variety in your diet. In order of best first, this is how forms of processing take away from an otherwise perfect food: juicing (fibre lost, but nutritional loss is minimal); dehydration under 48°C (only 2–5 per cent of nutrients lost, enzymes largely remain), freezing (5–30 per cent loss), steaming (up to 60 per cent); cooking (varies greatly depending on method, but basically the hotter the temperature, the worse the damage, so frying is at the highest end of the scale) – but nothing tops microwaving (90–99 per cent). Of all cooking methods, microwaving is the most potentially harmful as well as being a nightmare as far as nutrient loss is concerned. It operates in a very different way to traditional cooking. Instead of heating up from the outside, it works by making the food molecules vibrate so fast that this produces heat through friction at an alarming speed. As you can imagine, it completely throws the food's integrity out of balance and renders it a poor and very dysfunctional shadow of its former self.[19]

At the other end of the scale, the most beneficial and potent of all foods are a class of raw foods known as 'living foods'. So called because they are literally still growing and therefore 'alive', these foods are positively teeming with first-class living nutrition. Their vitality becomes self-evident in the way they look with their fresh strong shoots and through the way you feel when you eat them. Plus, they taste delicious!

Types of foods falling into this category are all sprouted foods such as seeds, beans, pulses, nuts and grains, soaked sea vegetables (rehydration reconstitutes them) and the grow-your-own greens such as sunflower greens, buckwheat 'lettuce' and wheatgrass (for juicing only).

You can read about how to grow these in Chapter 7.

Frequently asked questions

Cooked food in a cold climate

Another often-raised issue about raw-food eating is concerned with cold weather. 'I can understand that in summer eating raw foods must be wonderful,' people say, 'but what about in the winter? Surely we must need to eat hot foods? How can you possibly not want a bowl of hot soup?'

Left to its own devices, the body generates its own heat perfectly well, especially if more high-fuel raw foods are eaten such as nuts, dried fruits, certain herbs and spices and some of the more peppery leafy greens such as rocket. In the case of eating cooked/hot foods, the body is temporarily stimulated by the incoming heat and its temperature changes, but essentially the cooked food robs the system of energy, as we have seen, and it is not long before the body returns to its previous state. Eating raw food gives energy instead, thus freeing the body up to maintain a comfortable temperature permanently. We discovered ourselves that, over time, our need for and attraction to hot foods simply waned.

What about germs?

As so many health scares remind us, raw foods can be teeming with bacteria that can be potentially harmful unless destroyed with heat or other means. This is undoubtedly the case with raw animal products and processed foods, but far less likely with fresh fruit and vegetables. However, adequate washing of the produce along with clean storage and sensible personal hygiene are all vital whatever you eat. If you are away from home or are unsure of the hygiene of your food source, and especially if it is not organic, it is always wisest to peel your fruits and vegetables. In Chapter 7 we look at the toxins in raw beans and pulses and see how these are transformed in the sprouting process.

But remember, if you are healthier from eating a more vibrant diet and consequently have a stronger immune system, then you will be far better equipped to deal with any stray unfriendly bacteria, wherever it originates from.

The generations effect

'My gran ate cooked foods all her life and it never did her any harm.' This can be a common response. And indeed, the human body is an incredible surviving mechanism and will draw out all the available nutrition it can from whatever we eat. However, there is no doubt that there has been, and continues to be, a massive increase of chronic disease in our world, especially in the West where cancer and heart disease proliferate. Both of these are known to be, at least partly, diet-related. In fact, some scientists believe we should be living 120 years or more.

Some very poignant experiments were conducted in

the 1930s, by an American physician Francis Pottenger, Jr., to investigate the difference between animals fed on raw food and those fed on cooked food.[20] Pottenger began what was to become a ten-year diet study involving several hundred cats. What had started as a casual observation evolved into a meticulously controlled experiment which showed that with each progressive generation the ailments, diseases, malformations and even behavioural changes in the cats became more and more alarming.

He first began by splitting the cats off into two groups: one that was fed exclusively raw foods (their usual fare of meat, bones, milk and cod liver oil) and the other which consumed the same foods but with the meat cooked (in any number of ways, including boiling and frying) as typically fed to humans. He then very carefully observed and noted what happened to each group and their litters over the next few generations.

While those fed on the traditional fare of all raw foods maintained their health and vitality as they always had done, those fed the cooked meat products very quickly began to show incredibly disturbing changes:

First-generation 'cooked-food cats' (fed on cooked meat diet after maturity): heart problems, short- or long-sightedness, thyroid problems, infections of major organs, arthritis and joint inflammations, inflammation of the nervous system with paralysis and meningitis.

Second-generation 'cooked-food cats' (litter of first generation): the above symptoms became progressively worse and, generally speaking, the litter was much more irritable and dangerous to handle. There was also a very real problem in the reproductive aspect of their health: 83 per cent of males produced no sperm and 53 per cent of females showed only primordial ova. The rate of miscarriage was around 70 per cent compared to 25 per cent in the first generation, and deliveries were generally difficult, with many mothers dying in labour. Likewise many kittens were either stillborn or too frail to nurse and died because of this.

Third-generation 'cooked-food cats' (litter of second generation): by this point the surviving cats were so weak and deficient that any kittens they did manage to produce did not live beyond six months.

No wonder present-day processed cat food has to contain a whole host of added nutrients to try and compensate for the damaging effects of the cooked meats they contain.

Further investigations showed that regeneration was possible, but it would take four generations to get back to normal, with a reduction in symptoms along the way. The most noted aspect of the experiment overall was the effect on facial bone structure, teeth and bones. The findings showed that those cats fed on the cooked diet developed structural abnormalities, poor tooth formation and high rates of infection and that bone density was severely compromised.

Of course, cats have very different digestive systems

to humans and what suits them isn't what suits us. Nevertheless, it is striking how a change from a raw – albeit meat – diet to a cooked diet so dramatically affected their health.

Other food concerns

There are some processed foods, cooked or otherwise, which are especially bad for your health and should be avoided when rediscovering your intuition.

Caffeine and other stimulants

One cup of coffee typically contains between 70 and 120mg of caffeine: if this amount of caffeine was injected straight into your bloodstream it would kill you.[21] This beautifully illustrates how stimulating substances work. Basically caffeine is a poison and the body needs to go into 'fast-action' mode in order to clear the substance out quickly. This speeding-up of the system can feel wonderful as it gives one the illusion of having more energy and vitality, but sadly this is far from the truth. The whole process uses up valuable body resources such as minerals, therefore depleting our reserves further, and leading to less energy overall. Other foods which have this stimulating effect include meat products and alcohol.

Grain drugs

Most of us do not go a single day without some grain or cereal product passing our lips on at least one occasion.

Whether it's muesli, cereal, toast or sandwiches, pasta, rice or pizza, grains have become a national staple.

Although humans have been walking the planet for an estimated 2.5 million years, the harvesting and eating of grain is thought to have come into the equation only ten to twenty thousand years ago, clearly showing that we do not need grains at all in our diet to live healthily.

In fact, research into grain products has uncovered some worrying facts. Most notable are those studies that found opioid activity in wheat, maize and barley.[22] Opioids are drug-like substances known to quieten or deaden the mind or feelings. It is interesting to note that most common drugs of addiction are either opioid, such as heroin or morphine, or at the other end of the scale, dopaminergic, such as cocaine and amphetamine. No wonder a lot of people trying to give up wheat products have had quite a difficult time of it. Due to this opioid effect, bread is a typical example of a comfort food, something that many people use – albeit unconsciously – to slow themselves down.

If grains are neither necessary nor ideal foods for human consumption, in terms of holistic health it is far better to address the underlying problem that causes the need to use comfort foods. In the following chapter we detail how to recognise which need is making you want a certain type of food. What also should be taken into account is the acidifying effect of these foods, as mentioned earlier – the grain might calm you, but it also robs you of your mineral and enzyme reserves!

Optimum nutrition

Vibrant health is a natural state – again, look to nature and see that energy, vitality, enthusiasm, litheness and ease are very much the norm, in both adults and children. From birth, good health is the starting-point for the majority of us and as we mature we can either build on and utilise it or we can turn away from it by eating and drinking inappropriately and acting in other health-compromising ways. It's really no wonder that health and vitality decrease as we get older – and yet this is considered a 'normal' consequence of ageing.

Whether we are aware of it or not, the body is constantly going all out to maintain the best possible level of health. It speaks to us in a multitude of ways, from the odd headache (for example) or an outbreak of eczema, to life-threatening conditions such as cancer. The more hazardous our inner situation becomes, the louder the warning signals. What makes all the difference is how quickly we as individuals recognise and act on them.

Here is some serious food for thought from Ann Wigmore, the famous living foods pioneer who co-founded the Hippocrates Health Institute in America:

The best method in dealing with cancer problems is first to remove the cause. A diet containing uncooked nourishment will help to cleanse and rebuild the cells into a healthy state ... The most thrilling experience I can recall was seeing cancer cells taken from a human body thriving on cooked food, but unable to survive on food when it was uncooked. Such an experience taught me something that textbooks and teachers never can erase from my mind. For the human body, an uncooked vegetarian diet is the *only* type of nutrition.[23]

When assessing our own overall health, diet is of course only part of a very large picture. It is no good eating a great diet and then not looking after your emotional health, for example. Environmental factors cannot be ignored either, although they might be harder to deal with. This is another reason why our focus throughout this book is to encourage you to maintain awareness of your holistic well-being. Nevertheless, the food we eat is as important a place to start as any.

Food and the bigger picture

Eating in tune with our body, which means natural unprocessed foods, as direct from the plant, tree or bush as possible, automatically means that we are going to be eating more harmoniously for the planet as a whole. Apart from the obvious savings in terms of healthcare, medical prescriptions, time off work and the improvement of our quality of life in general, just think of the packaging, waste and pollution that could be avoided! Visit any landfill site and you will see for yourself just how much plastic, cardboard, polystyrene and so on we routinely throw away without a second thought, and how detrimental our eating habits are to the environment alone. How many of us would rethink our consumption of such environmental nightmares if we had to dispose of our own rubbish, rather than relying on our reliable refuse collector. By eating mainly, or totally, raw foods you can dramatically decrease the amount of rubbish you generate, finding that a small kitchen bin and a bucket for compost (peelings, pulp from juicing, skins and seeds etc) can be all you need to take care of your kitchen waste. And of course, by adding the compost to the soil, you'll be enriching it rather than polluting it, thus continuing the natural cycle and order of things.

As we discuss in Chapter 7, the best-case scenario is obviously growing your own fruit and vegetables and picking them straight from your garden or neighbourhood, thus eating locally grown produce. The next best is to buy from an organic farmers' market or wholefood warehouse where manpower, distribution and other energy costs are kept to a minimum. The further away from these we get, the bigger the implications both to ourselves and to the environment.

The subject of imported foods, especially tropical fruits, is a problematic issue for intuitive eaters. It is true that a great deal of energy and money is expounded on airfreighting in fresh produce which, much of the time, is really unfit for consumption anyhow, being picked underripe. But it is also true that many of these, when harvested organically or tree-ripened, can be a delicious and nutritious food source and can bring a lot of variety to a raw-food diet. Do whatever feels right for you – perhaps allow yourself the freedom to try new things, but also allow your conscience the airplay it needs. The importance of being honest with yourself does not end at just reading your body signals!

Anyone following global issues will know that historically we are at a very critical time. Obviously this book is written for those of us in the affluent Western world who are fortunate enough to have a great deal of choice and yet often have no real understanding of the way our choices affect those in the poorer nations. Consumerism has increased so dramatically over the past 50 years that it hardly bears thinking about. While creating comfort and luxury for some, affluence has encouraged greed and led to severe deprivation and exploitation for others sharing this planet. Typically, we own more than we make use of, we buy more than we need, we eat more than we require. Simplifying your life can be one of the most refreshing and freeing things you ever did.

Simplifying your diet brings similar rewards. You feel cleaner, fresher, new. You have a sense of possibility, the fog begins to lift, you can see things more clearly and objectively.

In 1986, after suffering for several years with chronic fatigue syndrome and candidiasis, I discovered the power of a healthy diet. I started to consume an increasingly high-percentage raw, vegan diet, and went all-raw in 1991. My health went from miserable to an incredibly high level within a year. Headaches, sinus infections, food allergies, candidiasis, all disappeared, and have yet to return. I experience more energy than I ever thought possible, and am often told how healthy I look.

Loren Lockman, USA

3 Contacting our Own Inner Wisdom

I knew after my first two raw days that the various drugs, allergy and blood tests, elimination diets and invasive procedures to find the 'cause' of my chronic irritable bowel had been a complete waste of time. All I had to do was listen to my body, then put two and two together. I feel like a truly different person – and I'm still near the beginning of my journey.

Sara Shooter, UK

Inner messages

Each time we think about food there are a whole range of inner voices that give us different messages about what action to take. Our intuition is our inner wisdom, the part of us that can listen to all of these voices and work out what we can do to best fulfil our needs.

Even though our intuition may have lain dormant for years, perhaps since very early childhood, we all still have access to its help and direction. This chapter and the next describe techniques that will enable you to re-discover your inner guide and make eating the pleasure it was originally designed to be.

Step one on this journey is to learn inner awareness. Just what happens inside us when the subject of food enters our head? What are the individual voices that talk to us through our thoughts and feelings?

To illustrate just how many differing messages we receive from ourselves, imagine it is 1 pm and you are in a crowded high street, with about half an hour free. Do any of these thoughts sound familiar to you?

'Hey, it's lunchtime, I'd better eat something now 'cause I won't get a chance later.'

'I heard that the new deli sells wonderful pasties, perhaps I'll try one.'

'Oh no, I can't do that, the garlic's far too strong, no one will want to come near me all afternoon.'

'Mmm, that bakery smells wonderful, maybe I'll have a baguette instead.'

'Oh yes – then I can buy some of that gorgeous cheese spread they keep advertising on the TV.'

'But that's too fattening – what else can I have?'

'Maybe I need some fish 'cause I'm getting those white flecks in my nails again. Perhaps I'm protein-deficient, or maybe it's not enough calcium.'

'But fishpaste just reminds me of school dinners and that's the last thing I want today.'

'Okay, how about a chocolate cream pie? Scrummy – and naughty.'

'But I keep on being "naughty", it's got to stop now.'

'Anyway I've spent far too much already on food this week, so I need something cheap, healthy and quick.'

'So how about a boring salad sandwich?'

'Ugh! I'd rather go hungry. Oh well, maybe I'm not *that* hungry. I just don't know – I've got too much to do anyway. Perhaps I'll grab something later.'

Sound familiar? We are constantly bombarded with these tiny voices in our minds, as well as all the inputs from our senses: smell, touch, taste, sight and sound. It's no wonder we're often confused and end up going from one extreme choice to the next.

These inner messages can be seen as arising from some basic categories, many of which we discuss below. None of them carry more importance than any of the others, however, so therefore they are all valued individually and equally in the intuitive process, as we shape our decisions about what to eat and why.

Physical needs

So how well do you know your physical body? The previous chapter described the key elements that the scientific researchers have so far discovered to be necessary for a 'healthy' diet. Luckily our body is already aware of these nutrients and gives us clear physical signals when it is low in any of them, such as fats, proteins, sugars, or vitamins and minerals.

However, we rarely need just one element at a time, so our body will give us signals for a variety of things, often all at once. Also nutrients work together for greater assimilation – for instance, we need magnesium and vitamin D for calcium absorption, but even then too much magnesium, zinc, phosphorus and even excessive exercise can hinder our uptake of calcium.

But don't panic! The beauty of eating intuitively is that, at an intellectual level, you don't need to understand all the possible signals your body may give you when it needs a particular nutrient, or has too much of it. You don't need to know which elements go with which for optimum assimilation, or what to avoid for blocking some nutrient's absorption and which food contains what. Your body knows this already. You just have to watch your body and get to know your own signs, so that you can gradually begin to tell the difference between a craving for something because you have an unhealthy addiction to it, or perhaps because you have an emotional need to fill, and a genuine craving for a specific nutrient that you are in need of at the time.

As you return to the diet your body was designed for, the signals start to become incredibly clear, and consequently it isn't long before you can begin to trust your instincts again.

Physical addictions

As we mentioned earlier, not only are tobacco, alcohol and various recreational drugs addictive, but so too are many cooked and processed foods that behave in similar biochemical ways. Naturally this condition greatly affects our food choices.

Heating raw plant foods to cooking temperatures brings about molecular changes and these can cause addictive and even allergic reactions in our bodies. For example, some people have an allergy or sensitivity to cooked wheat products; however they often have no problems with raw sprouted wheat. We are also often victims of the sugar or salt buzz – the stimulating effect of a lot of processed foods. In fact, it has been found that for many people with food intolerances, sensitivities and allergies, the foods they crave and feel they need most are often the very ones that they are most allergic or sensitive to. Therefore, how can we possibly trust our instincts with regard to these foods?

Obviously, products to which you can get subtly addicted mean big business for the food producers – what better way to ensure that their customers keep on returning to their products? Bear in mind that many foods available in our stores haven't just been heat-treated, but much of the time have also been fractured, reconstituted, 'enriched' and completely changed from their original state.

Social needs

Most of us belong to a social group made up of family, friends, work colleagues and the wider community within our home town, county or nation. To satisfy our sense of belonging, many of us need to share some aspects of each other's lifestyles. For others, this social need works the other way: these individuals want to be different from everyone else so they actively reject some of the key practices of those around them. In all cultures food-sharing is a key part of social interaction. Food turns up constantly in our social lives, from going out for a meal with friends, to the family Sunday dinner, to sharing a box of popcorn at the cinema, or even giving chocolates on Valentine's Day.

Fear of becoming a social outcast, or simply of being seen as awkward because of our dietary preferences will often make us compromise our real food needs and eat things we would really rather not. For instance, how many people do you suppose eat those small slices of over-sugared birthday or wedding cakes just because of tradition (and because everyone else does) instead of genuinely liking the product? The same goes for the customary cup of tea and coffee or the soft or alcoholic drink almost always offered at social occasions. If everyone else has a cup or a glass in their hands we tend to feel out of place if we decline the offer of one.

Social situations can also conjure up other food reactions, so that we might eat a lot more or a lot less than we would at home. For example, if, as a child, you were part of a large family and food was limited, as an adult at a dinner party you might find yourself unconsciously eating quickly to be sure of a second helping before anyone else. This could mean that you end up eating far more than perhaps you have a real appetite for.

Conditioning influences

We are born and grow up within a particular lifestyle, with certain routines and habits. These get imprinted in what is termed our 'psychological conditioning' and can influence our feelings of being comfortable with our present adult lifestyle.

For instance, if you always have three meals a day, it could prove uncomfortable to miss out on even one meal for a sustained period. Or if your mother had been very concerned about whether you were getting enough protein as a child, this could become an out-of-proportion concern in your own food choices as an adult, or in your choices for your children.

These tendencies also emerge strongly at times of psychological or emotional difficulties. For example, if you were always offered sweets or treats when you were upset as a child, this may be what you will crave at similar times as an adult. You could also find yourself craving favourite childhood foods in times of stress or when you are at a loss over what to eat.

Having large meals at set times of the day is another extremely common pattern in our culture. Imagine eating just when you are really hungry, and just the right amount to satisfy that hunger – instead of leaving the table feeling stuffed or sleepy because the body needs a lot of energy to digest the meal. Does this sound possible?

Self-esteem

Lack of self-esteem is a virulent disease in our culture and we all carry a version of it. Even the seemingly most confident person often nurses secret feelings of not being good enough.

Do you find it difficult to do things that are pleasurable just for you? When was the last time you bought yourself a present or did something completely selfish? 'Selfishness' is almost an insulting word in our language because it gives the impression that to be selfish you don't care about anyone else. However, to be truly selfish means the opposite. If you have learnt the ultimate care – ie to be able to care for and respect yourself – you will then have a massive capacity to be able to care genuinely for others.

It is those who *do not* care for themselves who display the most destructive 'selfish' behaviour because they treat others as, deep down they really treat themselves (on the surface, such people may exhibit very greedy tendencies but this is only a façade). To be healthily 'selfish' is to feed yourself on every level so that you are fuelled up to feed others even more.

Lack of self-esteem also leads to feelings of unworthiness which can result in all sorts of food messages, such as emotional comfort-eating, starvation, or simply feeling as if we are not worth the effort of buying and preparing a nutritious meal for.

How many of us are unhappy with the way we look and feel, or how we perceive others to view us? Our culture is saturated with the knock-on effects of the weight-loss industry, which thrives on people feeling too fat and unhappy with their appearance. When we dwell on this, eating can become a nightmare of calorie counting and guilt bingeing and it is possible that some kind of obsession with food can develop which is blown completely out of proportion. With such a mindset, could you eat three avocados in a meal without a niggling voice in the back of your head telling you how fattening they are, and how every mouthful is adding inches to your waist?

Alongside the weight-loss industry sits the body-building business which feeds on the concerns of those who feel they are too skinny and therefore must eat good 'solid' food and follow muscle-building programmes in order to fill out and gain weight.

These neuroses are continually compounded by the media, who tell us what is perfect or normal. These vital statistics are often unattainable for the majority of the population, leading to deep dissatisfaction, low self-esteem and often eating disorders, which in turn lead to serious weight and health problems.

So food may carry many other priorities besides satisfying hunger and physical need. Our heads may be asking, 'How many calories? Will it fill me up enough? Is this good or bad food?' Does this sound familiar?

Emotional eating

A classic example of emotional eating is reaching for a chocolate bar when we are experiencing difficult feelings, such as sadness, anger or even ecstasy. If, for instance, you are going through a very stressful, fearful time in your life, the emotions that arise inside may unconsciously seem too big to handle, and eating can become a brilliant way of not allowing these to be fully felt. It's almost like an emotional switching-off. To find out why these emotions can feel overwhelming, it is necessary to return to our childhood to see why we have never learnt to handle them.

In our society, many children do not have the opportunity to fully experience and express their emotions. The standard adult response is to 'protect' the child from 'difficult' feelings, perhaps because the adult finds these too painful to witness, having buried their own emotions many decades ago. It is often an unconscious response to cajole a child to stop crying, or to exclaim, 'Stop making that awful noise' even when there is something to scream about. Children who aren't permitted this freedom of expression learn to keep their emotions to themselves, bottling them up inside. As aware as parents try to be, it is often still the case that boys are taught not to cry, and girls are not allowed to express anger.

Many of us have therefore learnt ways of switching off our strong uncomfortable feelings. Common ways of doing this can be:

- by being very busy, thereby avoiding having the time to feel
- by being very social or engaging in activities of which the focus remains external
- by 'blanking off' through watching television, reading a book, or listening to music
- by taking mind/body changing substances such as alcohol, cigarettes or drugs
- by eating 'comfort-foods' or practising self-starvation to take our minds off our feelings.

'Comfort foods' will mean different things to each individual. Some will need the tranquillising effect of bread and heavy cooked starches, while others will need the zapping effect of sugars and other stimulants such as coffee and chocolate.

Inertia and fear of change

This can prevent us from experimenting with foods that are unfamiliar and are therefore seen as risky. Our inner voice may say:

'What if this way of eating doesn't work?'
'What if I have even less energy?'
'What if my children complain?'
'But I love my current food, I couldn't change that!'
'But I have no time to work out anything new.'

Have you also found that you get more fearful as you grow older? Do you feel that there are many things which you would have happily tackled as a teenager, but which now fill you with unjustified apprehension?

Even though our current way of eating causes problems and has worrying consequences, making changes to something as fundamental as the food that sustains us can prove very difficult, unless we have the support of our family and friends. Indeed, it often seems to take masses of energy to put a new idea into practice. But just as a large boulder takes a lot of effort to set it in motion, it gathers momentum as it rolls along and soon no effort is required at all.

Advice and influence of others

We are constantly being offered the advice and opinions of others. Whether this be from doctors, nutritionists, naturopaths, teachers, friends, family, or the media, we are taught from a very early age that there is always someone else who knows better than us and whose opinions are more valuable than our own. Likewise, given half a chance, we are all keen to get our own perspective across to those in need!

Most of the time, the advice we receive from others is well meaning and often well informed, but how much of it is influenced by the other person's individual experiences, their own possible prejudices and hidden intentions? For example, a friend may advise you about the merits of a new health cure because they are about to try it for themselves and are unconsciously looking for someone to try it with them for moral support. Or perhaps an unscrupulous healthcare practitioner may recommend a particular remedy to you because it means more profit for them.

Not only are we subjected to the constant opinions of others, we are almost suffocated by advertising – it's everywhere! As well as the obvious sources such as television, newspapers and magazines, the products of advertisers subtly permeate our psyches in all sorts of unlikely places, such as when driving along the road, or pulling up behind a bus – you can even find advertisements on the backs of parking permits!

Notice, too, how retail outlets use clever positioning of their products and display them in attractive packaging to catch our eye. Some supermarkets even pipe the aroma of freshly baked bread to entice us to buy specific foods. Do you suppose as much fresh meat would be sold if the product was not sealed away by being wrapped up in plastic, or if the shop smelt like the abattoir where the meat came from?

The concern here is that one generation of disempowered adults will naturally lead to subsequent generations of yet more disempowered adults with little belief in themselves and even less knowledge about how to improve their own situation.

Food availability

Our food choices are limited by what we can obtain from shops or grow and gather ourselves. There is also the financial consideration to be taken into account. It is important to acknowledge here that our government subsidises many products to maintain the current political status quo. Perhaps eating habits would change if bread and dairy products were not the heavily subsidised industries that they are today.

A raw, intuitive diet need not be expensive. By purchasing locally grown products and growing a proportion of your food yourself (no garden needed – see the section on sprouting in Chapter 7) – such a way of eating can often be much cheaper than the standard British diet (not to mention more enjoyable, fulfilling, nutritious and healthy!).

All our inner voices are vital

Bundle all these messages together, and it's no wonder that the whole eating game can seem like a minefield. If we are craving a particular food, which inner voice is asking for it? How do we tell the voices apart and which ones should affect our final choices? How long is it going to take to decide what to eat each time we feel like food? Life would obviously be very complicated if we had to analyse everything we thought, felt and saw, so thankfully there is a better way.

This is where the deployment of our intuition is vital. It will do all of this work for us. Do we have to think about taking each breath? Do we need to worry that perhaps there is not enough oxygen around, or that our lung capacity might not be adequate, every time we breathe? Luckily for the vast majority of us, there is an automatic unconscious function that takes care of all this and the same can be true for food choices. We all have a completely natural function which takes into account, and values, *all* our needs, and not just our nutritional requirements, without any conscious planning or thought on our part.

The first vital step to take is in the realisation that all these inner needs are part of us and therefore of the greatest importance to our everyday lives. They need to be acknowledged for what they are and not disowned, buried or ignored.

Just because we may, for example, find ourselves heavily influenced by the eating habits of our friends, which may be contrary to our real food desires, this doesn't mean that we are weak willed or inferior. It is important to value that aspect of ourselves and to take into account the fact that social needs are important to us and need to be honoured in some way.

If needs and feelings are ignored and we pretend they don't exist, then they will never go away. Instead they will eventually throw a spanner into the works of any idealised, intellectualised eating plan that we try to follow using will-power alone. If, for example, we were to pretend that we weren't going to be influenced by the eating habits of our friends, we would probably start to feel very isolated and lonesome – which could lead to comfort-eating the sorts of foods that we didn't even want anyway!

So, all our inner needs require to be heard, acknowledged and respected by us, so that we can work with them, rather than ignore them in the vain hope that something magic will happen and our cravings for 'inappropriate' foods will disappear overnight. When you are working with your intuition, valuing and honouring your whole self, you will be amazed at how creative you can be in finding constructive solutions to 'problems' that have been around for years. If, for example, you have been overeating for comfort since childhood, you could well find many more effective ways of looking after these comfort needs once the intuitive process has deepened your self-respect.

You will find, as you begin to modify your diet, that your various food needs and cravings often have very deep roots and can't be changed with good intentions alone. For example, do calorie counters ever really lose their desire for chocolate or chips? Will-power may have its benefits, but it can never irrevocably change our habits since mind-over-matter without the backing of genuine feelings is only a recipe for discomfort. The key to success, therefore, is self-acceptance and forgetting the guilt trips. Only then can new ways come in and lifetime habits really disappear.

How to practise inner awareness

As explained earlier, to initiate your intuitive abilities you need to begin by gaining skills in self-observation. Observation is the key term here, not necessarily understanding or analysing each inner message. We live in a very intellectual culture, in which we are encouraged to understand our feelings instead of just experiencing them. By becoming more aware of your inner processes – by allowing your feelings, not thinking about them or asking *why?* – your intuition is freed up to work for you. Consequently your self-respect increases and, with it, your self-esteem, and life has the potential to get a whole lot better, more satisfying and more constructive.

Before you begin

1 Raising your self-esteem

You need to have a deep sense of self-worth to help you self-improve or heal destructive habits, so the first vital step in this process of self-discovery is to achieve a healthier level of self-esteem. The mere fact that you are reading this book means you have an interest in self-help, so your self-esteem is not completely rock bottom!

There are many books and tapes available detailing ways of enhancing your self-esteem. We have found that guided visualisations and positive affirmations really work. Ask for information at your local library or bookstore.

2 Creating space

As mentioned previously, being busy is a wonderful excuse for not actually changing anything. Often we can feel completely swamped by the number of things we have to do in a day. It can feel as if there just isn't the time to think, let alone to make changes or sit still and relax. We buy time-saving machines, only to fill the consequent spare time with more activities and responsibilities.

Our culture supports this busyness syndrome in that the busier you make your life the more successful you are seen as being. Yet frantically going from one activity to the next, amassing stress and scrambling one's thoughts, ultimately never leads to greater success – instead it usually ends up with us chasing our own tails, fraught with anxiety and fatigue. Those who achieve the greatest 'success' tend to be those who make time in their lives for stillness, for inner contemplation, and who have a more relaxed attitude to the way they address their lives. Because they are less frantic they are better able to prioritise their activities, successfully judging which ones are not really necessary.

To be able to practise self-observation we need to STOP for brief periods each day just to be able to watch ourselves, instead of trying to *do, do, do.*

Learning to stop and self-observe could unconsciously seem like a frightening prospect. However, intellectually we can comfort ourselves with the realisation that we learnt that fear of experiencing our emotions as young children, when emotions were more powerfully experienced because they were new and unknown and generally not fully allowed. As adults, this fear is generally no longer justified as we are far better equipped to fully experience these feelings.

Naturally, for some, there will be times when very difficult past memories and emotions are uncovered which might feel overwhelming. In these circumstances it is very important to look after yourself and seek support from an appropriate health practitioner, counsellor or therapist who will be able to help you heal some of the past.

When you create brief periods of stillness in your busy day you will be amazed at the difference in the way you feel and view yourself and your life. In addition to releasing your intuitive abilities, positive qualities will emerge such as greater self-confidence, a more relaxed attitude, and more of a will to sort out how you really want to live your life.

3 Checking your attitude

The way we approach our day has an immense effect on the quality of our experience. For example, if stuck in a traffic jam, you have two basic choices about how you feel. First (and most common) you could feel stressed, full of worry and impatience, perhaps even angry and irritable, and you could end up cursing all the surrounding drivers, the police, or those who have caused the delay. The other option is to be grateful for the situation because it allows you time to relax, to put some good music on the stereo, and just to enjoy the space and time available. Of course it's the same traffic jam, but two very different attitudes leading to very differing potential experiences of your day. Which would you prefer?

Although we have a tendency to moan and fret about our lives, it is usually possible to see the silver lining in any scenario and, because our initial attitudes colour everything we experience and feel, to have a lighter, less stressful existence.

Steps to practising self-observation

Stage 1 – General inner observation

For this you need to have regular time alone with yourself, with no other agendas going on. Perhaps you need to put on the answerphone, tell the family that you're out of communication for a while, or wait until young children are asleep before you start your 'watching time'.

This need only take about ten minutes a day at first, and can slowly increase with practice. It can become quite alluring if you rarely have time alone just to 'be'.

With this space to yourself, all you have to do is NOTHING. Sit comfortably, and just watch your thoughts and feelings – it's as simple as that.

Find a time when you are not overtired and find a comfortable, alert sitting position so that you are not encouraging yourself to drop off to sleep!

At first you may spend your time thinking about anything and everything as different thoughts just wander in and out. The trick is not to get stuck on one particular thing but to develop a sense of detachment from the actual subjects, so that eventually you will feel like an outside observer watching yourself think. You will find that the thoughts are like clouds racing across a blue sky – they just come and go.

Similarly, many emotions can also surface and you may find yourself spontaneously laughing or crying as the sensations wash over you.

To develop this ability to observe your thoughts and feelings without getting caught up in them, try any of the following basic focusing exercises:

1 Find a comfortable sitting position and close your eyes. Take a few deep, long breaths just to start relaxing the body and to make it comfortable. Begin the exercise by watching the rise and fall of your breathing rhythm and then, after a few breaths, allow any thoughts or feelings to wander in. If you find yourself suddenly miles away and well into a thought train, gently bring yourself back to watching your breathing for a few breaths. Then allow it to wander again briefly, before bringing it gently back to the breath again and again.

2 Repeat the above exercise, but choose something visual to focus your attention on, to keep you from wandering off too far into a thought stream. One way to do this is by sitting comfortably in front of a blank wall and gently focusing the eyes along the bottom of the wall. This way your eyes are half closed, and each time the mind wanders, you can gently bring your attention back to the wall.

3 While sitting comfortably alone with no distractions, write down everything that goes through your mind in a ten-minute session – even thoughts like 'I'm feeling stupid doing this' if that's what's going on at the time. You'll be amazed at the thoughts that do pass through.

4 The trick here is to speak your thoughts into a tape recorder to make a record of all those voices that wander in and out of your mind. Some people are

even able to talk directly to a 'listening' person in this way. However, this listening person needs to have quality passive listening skills in order to be able to give you their full attention, and not offer their own head chatter with their ideas, solutions, opinions or interpretations.

5 You can use arts and crafts, and any type of material such as paints, crayons, clay, sand etc, to allow the free expression of what you're feeling and thinking. For example, try making a frieze of your wandering thoughts, so that you record the differing voices in some way along each step of the frieze as they travel through your mind.

6 All manner of creative ways can be used to express what is going on at that very moment in your inner world. Some people use dance or other body movements, whereas others use sound, or songs or make up stories that reflect just what is going on inside their heads.

The important factor in all these exercises is to find a way that suits your individuality. The best approach for you is to find one you enjoy and are therefore more likely to want to follow on a daily basis. We all have our strengths and weaknesses so you need to ask yourself whether you are happiest visually, with sound, or with kinaesthetics (the sense of touch which could be deployed with clay etc).

The aim is to gain some space in your life to start experiencing your full self – not to understand all your voices, but to initiate the process of greater self-awareness. By starting with ten minutes a day of concentrated observation, you will gradually become more and more aware of your differing thoughts and needs throughout the day, even at your busiest times. Self-observation grows of its own accord once we have given it the space and the initial push.

It is essential to be non-judgemental with your thoughts during these times. Every thought and feeling is important and valid to you. If, for example, you find yourself thinking about how much you dislike your boss, and then blame yourself for being so full of contempt, you are in fact experiencing two inner voices: the first one is expressing a personal grievance against an authority figure, and the second exists just to give you a hard time for experiencing negative feelings towards others.

You may want to start extending this period of self-observation – not because we've told you it's good for you but because it's really what you want. Give yourself at least a month of a self-enforced quiet time of ten minutes daily, and then increase or decrease this according to your particular needs.

Naturally there are other positive side-effects to this daily time of self-contemplation. These include a deepening ability to relax and feel an inner calm, and to gain an increasing perspective on your everyday problems, with more clarity gradually spilling over into the rest of the day. However, do not allow this time alone to become an opportunity for focusing on problem-solving. It should be a time for unattached thoughts and observing your feelings without the need to analyse them or work things out.

Stage 2 – Food feelings

As you practise self-observation, at times your thoughts will naturally focus on foods. The next step is to develop this particular awareness in greater depth so that you are able to learn, on a deep, unconscious level, what feels good and what really doesn't work for you.

What happens in your thoughts and feelings each time you want to eat? Which voice is strongest, and where does it come from? Again it is really vital *not* to judge your feelings and get into guilt trips but just to be aware of them and accept them for what they are. If you fancy a chocolate bar, that's fine; it's not bad to want chocolate, it's just a part of you that needs it. This could be an addictive need, or perhaps a conditioning need, and all your needs are valid, as they are part of the rich tapestry of who you are.

With time, and by focusing on them, you will become aware of all your differing needs as they surface, such as social needs, or self-esteem needs, and others. Each time you eat, you don't need to ask yourself, 'Now why am I doing this?' Just watch the thoughts and experiences that accompany the food desires and eating processes and in time you will automatically know, not necessarily consciously, which need or mixture of needs you are fulfilling.

At this stage, and again for about a month, just watch yourself. You needn't try to alter your behaviour because of what you notice. So if, for example, you really want a plate of chips, go ahead and have them! But while you're eating you may want to reflect on exactly why you wanted them.

Self-awareness need not make food an obsession. At first there will be many mealtimes when you are not focusing your attention on your thoughts about food, and even when you are it is merely gentle observation – you needn't get into deep discussions with yourself about what's going on. Just watch, and your unconscious intuition will begin to do all the work. It will soon tell you if there is something you need to know.

Stage 3 – Going deeper

By now you will know yourself much better, and especially with regard to food, although of course you can apply this sort of awareness to any other area in your life to see what is really going on.

The next stage is to give yourself more raw food as an experiment to observe your 'inner feeling' reactions. Consult the information in the next chapter, along with recipes in Chapter 7, on how to gradually increase the percentage of raw food in your daily menus, and just watch how it all goes.

Also, try to simplify the foods you eat, such as strawberries without sugar and tomatoes without salt. Perhaps you need that condiment or tandem food to help mask a taste that your body doesn't like? If so, does it really make sense to disguise and then eat foods in this way? Some condiments, such as black pepper, actually have very toxic elements and could be damaging if eaten in any quantity.

After about a month of these eating changes, you may find it interesting to question yourself about which foods meet the criteria set by your different needs or, more specifically, whether each food is beneficial or detrimental to these needs. For example, you may find yourself craving a pizza for dinner because you think it will make you feel good, and it fits in with requests from the rest of your family. Beforehand you might revel in the aromas as it cooks, causing great salivation and anticipation. Once you bite in, however, you may discover that it doesn't quite live up to the promise of the smells; perhaps even after a large portion it doesn't feel 'enough' somehow, and possibly half an hour later you realise that it has left an odd aftertaste, and your stomach is feeling a bit uncomfortable.

All these types of observations would normally have gone unnoticed, so seeing them can be quite a revelation. Continue to watch these feelings, and maybe the recollection of what happened that time you ate the pizza will make the craving slightly less next time. This is the key to effortless change. You don't need to force yourself not to want pizza. All you have to do is to know what it really feels like to eat it and then, without even trying, you may find that eventually you don't really want pizza anymore.

So feasting on junk food and yo-yo-ing between healthier raw or cooked food need no longer be seen as a problem; in fact it is a positive advantage as it will give you lots more opportunities to deeply observe your differing reactions to a wide variety of foods. Through the skills of inner awareness, you will gradually develop solid inner wisdom about what foods really do work best for you.

Of course it is important to keep in perspective the addictive nature of cooked foods on the body and how our addictions can play such a strong role in our wanting certain foods, but as incredible as it may sound, even these can be easily overridden when you get more in tune with what you really want.

We were both amazed by our effortless ability to lose our well-entrenched chocolate addictions, but in time, with continual self-observation, and after eating a high raw diet, we came to find that it genuinely didn't taste good any more! After the initial two seconds' taste explosion we both, independently of each other, grew to really dislike the aftertaste of chocolate and how we felt for hours after eating it.

Perhaps surprisingly, self-observation soon develops into something that becomes an effortless part of your everyday life. It also gives you the wonderful freedom to follow your own truths about food. Your body, rather than other people, will be telling you what to eat and perhaps for the first time in years you will understand and respect it!

When this point is reached, foods will stop being 'good' or 'bad' because we all have differing lives and needs and what works for you might well not be right for someone else. Moreover, don't be surprised if your diet changes radically over the following months, because eating more raw food can often start a snowball effect. Chances are that once your body knows just how good raw foods feel compared to cooked foods it will want more and more of them!

4 Making Changes and What to Expect

This chapter goes into more detail about how to gradually increase the percentage of raw food in your diet and describes the sort of things you can expect to see in yourself.

If you have been observing your eating habits for a month, as suggested in Stage One of Chapter 3, perhaps ask yourself: 'How healthy am I right now? Where am I starting from?' If you have any serious health problems we recommend that you seek professional help and have the changes monitored by experts. We hope you will find the information in this book useful, but it must not replace seeking outside assistance if the need arises (see Useful Contacts). If, on the other hand, you consider your health to be reasonable, transferring to a more raw, intuitive diet should be relatively easy, as long as you take your time and allow things to happen naturally.

Begin by writing down some observations about yourself and the way you look and feel right now. Perhaps take some 'before' photos and jot down a few bodily measurements. Put all these in a journal so that you can look back in awe in a few months' time.

The detox test

As explored in Chapter 2, if we are clogged up on the inside, then our inner messages are bound to be confused. However, the good news is that by adopting a more raw diet for a few weeks, inner debris will start to cleanse out of your body.

Two very quick and easy ways to gauge your current inner state are the tongue test and the one-day detox. The tongue test officially begins after your lunchtime meal (or, at the latest, your mid-afternoon snack). After that, just for one evening, do not eat or consume anything but water. Then first thing next morning, go straight to the nearest mirror, stick out your tongue and take a good long look. You might be surprised! The chances are that what you will see is not the smooth pink tongue of yesterday morning after brushing your teeth, but instead a rather discoloured, furred-up version that you would gladly disown. Yellow or white? Thick coating or thin? Basically, what you have there is an indication of what is likely to be coating your colon and you can bet there's plenty more where that came from!

The one-day detox is not quite so blatant – you probably won't see the effects in the mirror, but you could well feel them in very real ways which the eye can't see. The key is to make it as easy and pleasurable for yourself as possible, so pick one juicy organic fruit which you really enjoy – from grapes, mangoes, apples, sweet oranges, papaya or melon. Avoid heavier fruits like bananas and avocados as these will not have the same effect (see the full list of lighter fruits in Chapter 7).

Choose a day when your workload is minimal, or you have time to relax if you want or need to, and then just eat that one fruit all day long – as much as you want, but only that one fruit (and drink plenty of water)... and then see what happens!

If you get through the day without cravings, headaches, feeling emotional or experiencing other uncomfortable symptoms, extend the mono eating for another day and see what happens then. The sooner you experience any discomfort, the more you are in need of a good cleansing! At this stage, restrict the detox test to just two days at the most and then slowly reintroduce other foods, keeping things simple and not using concentrated foods (otherwise known as low-water-content foods) such as dried fruits and nuts, for at least another day.

Once you have an idea of where you're starting from it will be much easier to gauge your progress so, again, be sure to write down as many details as you can at this early stage.

Step by step – how to introduce raw foods

When introducing raw foods some people like to dive in head first and use the 'all or nothing' approach. However, we recommend the gentler and more effective method of one small step at a time.

Thinking back to the natural cycles of the body, as outlined in Chapter 2, the easiest first step to take – and one which will help your body adjust to the transition – is the 'fruit for breakfast' rule where you can eat as much fruit as you desire but nothing else until lunchtime. If you're used to coffee and toast every morning then just add the fruit without taking anything away, but for ease of digestion do eat the fruit first and have the coffee and toast at least twenty minutes later. For those a little more used to this ideology, try swapping the coffee for freshly squeezed orange juice five mornings out of seven, or, if even that thought is too daunting, cut down on the number of sugars or sweeteners you're using and make the coffee weaker. There are many alternative breakfast suggestions in Chapter 7. At this stage, do whatever you can manage; however tiny the steps, just keep moving forward.

Next, start introducing more fresh foods into your lunchtime or evening meals – ideally both. This can be as simple as adding a modest side salad to each meal or replacing a cooked baked potato filling with, for example, mashed avocado, or perhaps a crunchy raw vegetable topping rather than a cooked spicy one. The variety, as you will see later, is practically endless. The main criterion is to eat as much food that is raw, fresh, and preferably *organic* as possible. And you needn't take away favourite processed foods, just add *more* raw ones!

Another key to intuitive eating is to make it fun and enjoyable. This is not a penance – it is your first step towards gastronomic heaven! So get creative and buy foods that you love. For example, if you usually eat sandwiches for lunch, buy some top-quality organic wholemeal pitta breads and fill them with anything fresh and as raw as you can manage – such as chunky slices of tomato and cucumber, crisp fresh lettuce and slivers of creamy avocado.

You can also replace those between-meal snacks with fruits, perhaps ones that you haven't tried before – experiment with papaya, mangoes, lychees, ugli fruit, blueberries and so on. Do be sure you get good advice from your grocer about whether these 'new' fruits are ripe, as it would be very sad if you were put off mangoes (for instance) just because you had tried a rock-hard, unripe one.

Also make sure you eat a good variety of foods within your week by experimenting with all sorts of ingredients. As you'll see in Chapter 7, there is such an incredible range of raw fruits and vegetables available to us that meal preparation can be as simple or as complex as we desire.

Cleansing

As the raw part of your diet increases, it won't be long before you begin to realise that something is definitely going on. It may start with a change as simple, but none the less gratifying, as an increase in energy or feeling happier in yourself. As the days turn to weeks, you may find yourself more alert on waking, thinking more clearly, feeling more balanced in your emotions and making positive food choices without thinking about them so much. You may also start to see more 'physical' signs such as your skin tone changing, spots clearing up, nails becoming stronger, breath being somewhat sweeter in the morning and, depending on your current body shape, tone and lift beginning to show.

With positive changes like these taking place, you could well find that you want to continue the process longer than a few weeks and this is when the experience really begins to offer life-changing possibilities. You could well find yourself looking in the mirror one day and thinking that you're looking younger than when you first started eating this way. Not just that, but you've lost many of those extra pounds, your eyes are cleaner and have more sparkle, and your hair and nails are stronger and shinier than perhaps ever before. And it probably won't end there – quite a few other curious things may have started happening. For example, you may have very little interest in eating junk foods, and if you do, you'll feel awful physically when you've indulged. You may also find that you don't have to use as much deodorant as before, or that you might forget to brush your teeth every now and again because the bad taste you used to get first thing in the morning has been missing lately. And don't be surprised if your toilet habits have changed either – you may find that your bowel movements are more regular than they have been for years.

Cleansing reactions

Along the way, it's true, you will have challenges. No journey worth making is an easy ride, and equally, neither is it boring! Obstacles and hurdles are unavoidable, so best be prepared for them. As long as you have some idea of what to expect, surmounting them will be so much easier.

The term 'detoxing' has become something of a buzzword during recent years. 'Detox in a weekend' and other equally appealing headlines appear in newspapers, books and magazines, making us believe that what took decades to accumulate can simply be lost in a matter of days. If only! The truth is that it will take quite some time to detoxify your body of all the debris stored up over the years and, because of the way the body works, it won't all happen in one go. 'Debris' includes pesticides, herbicides, fungicides, additives, preservatives, salt, sugar, junk fats, inappropriate chemicals and all other inorganic substances injected or ingested either through the food you've eaten or the air you've breathed – effectively anything your body does not recognise as fuel.

Detoxification is not known for being an ecstatic experience – or at least not at first – but it needn't be awful either. If you compare the human body to a river, we are born with a relatively clean and free-flowing internal system and life in such a body can be a real joy. Remember how you felt as a child, when running and playing were the norm and you barely knew your body was there? That terrific feeling of oneness, where the body was lithe and up for anything, need not be a thing of the past.

As the body begins to clog up – with the passing of time and as a result of ingesting less than optimum fuel – a few problems might start to show themselves. In the early days these can be as simple as colds, sore throats, ear infections and the like, which, traditionally, we keep at bay by resorting to outside measures such as medicines. We are surprised when these complaints return again and again, yet all the while we continue to do the same things and eat in the same way as we have always done. All the while the river that is our body is becoming more polluted and functioning less well. At some point, if the blockages become too significant, we may opt for surgery to remove the offending item. However, this is treating the symptoms and not the cause.

So when someone begins detoxification – and this means stopping, or at least reducing the amount of debris they are consuming – the body tends to take advantage of the situation. Suddenly, after eating in a new, cleaner way, people begin to experience unusual symptoms, or at least symptoms that they didn't expect. These can range from an upset stomach to a sore throat, to what feels like flu or a heavy cold, or maybe headaches, dizziness or even nightmares. When such things happen it is natural to be concerned and to wonder what's going on. It is simply nature taking its course and thanking you (although it may not feel like it) for making the effort to help. It's rather as if it has decided to make hay while the sun shines.

If, for any reason, you find some symptoms worrying and you don't feel altogether sure about what's taking place, do get your doctor or health practitioner to check you over for reassurance.

One reaction to detoxing symptoms we often hear is: 'How can I be feeling so bad if it's not the food doing it to me?' Certainly, at first, you may wonder whether your new diet is beneficial, but thinking things through logically, how could such clean, wholesome foods be any worse for you than all the processed, cooked foods you may have previously eaten? Quite simply, the cleansing symptoms are the evidence of what 'inappropriate' food creates inside. The streaming colds, upset stomachs, headaches and spots show you quite clearly exactly what your old diet has been storing up for years.

Cleansing – which way is out?

When the body begins to house-clean it makes use of all possible exits, which is why the kinds of symptoms you may experience can be very wide-ranging. As much as we would all like detoxification symptoms not to happen, they are helping us enormously to become much healthier and have more energy, so could almost be celebrated. When you begin cleansing your system, you will see the reality of what your particular 'river' has been harbouring for months, years, or even decades.

It would be impossible to list the complete range of possible detoxing reactions. Most people find that they have just one or two major symptoms, usually in a part of their body where they have had problems in the past. Our own experiences were of sporadic and spontaneous cleanses which felt like flu but were in some ways quite different. All in all, our detoxification was – and continues to be – relatively painless and gentle, with minimal impact on our lives.

The bloodstream

If debris – such as fat deposits – are leaving their old lodging sites then the first route out is generally through the bloodstream. Obviously they can then go on to exit via other elimination organs such as the skin or digestive system, but once in the bloodstream they can lead to various symptoms such as headaches, negative thoughts or generally 'feeling under the weather'. Also, it is usually when toxins are in the blood that food cravings make themselves felt.

The skin

The skin is the body's largest eliminative organ and as such the body will use this unreservedly to throw out toxins. This can take the form of anything from tiny spots to full-blown rashes or even boils, or sometimes just random itchy patches or dry areas.

You can assist the skin in its job by skin brushing with a specially made plant bristle brush available from chemists and shops like The Body Shop. The action of the brush helps to clear away dead cells and other eliminated toxins from the surface of the skin. You can also help your skin by using as few toiletries as possible. Some women find that wearing foundation on their face begins to cause problems as it blocks pores and therefore prevents skin elimination, adding further to the incoming workload. However, as your skins begins to rejuvenate itself you could well end up not wanting to wear anything on it anymore because you look healthy without it.

Eyes and ears

Our eyes and cars are less commonly used exits, but none the less, if you find yourself waking up with excess 'sleep' in your eyes you can bet that something's made its way out which didn't belong in there. We have both found that we now only get the tiniest amount of 'sleep' in our own eyes upon waking, if anything at all. Likewise for ears: you may find yourself needing to clean your ears more regularly at first as hardened wax can begin to soften and move towards being eliminated.

Nose

The chances are that every time you have a 'cold' you end up blowing your nose constantly. The nose is a great exit for mucus which fulfils the vital role of collecting any loosened inner debris needing urgent elimination, and carrying it quickly and easily out of the body.

Mouth

There are many books that elaborate on how the tongue is a mirror of the colon, and the tongue test mentioned on page 96 is one example of how you can see on the outside what's going on inside you. As you progress, do not be surprised if you begin to find yourself bringing up mucus in your mouth akin to that you blow out of your nose when you have a heavy cold. Although a bit alarming at first, this is an excellent way of ridding your body of an enormous amount of toxins in a very quick and concentrated way. It's not pretty, but it is what's going on inside you, so far better out than in!

Also your breath may fluctuate widely between

'normal' and foul as your digestive system cleans itself through.

Sweat glands

Did you ever wonder why sweat often smells so bad? Well, the truth is it doesn't have to. Many people who have adopted a purer vegetarian diet have found that they no longer have any need for antiperspirants or deodorants. The reality is that in a 'cleaner' (on the inside) body, sweat is not offensive but rather lightly fragranced or even unnoticeable. Whatever the smell of your body odour, you can bet it's a true reflection of your inner condition. Apart from the fact that many antiperspirants contain aluminium, which is thought to be extremely toxic to the body, they also inhibit natural elimination. Rather than focusing on masking or preventing our sweat, our attention should be turned to taking action to make it naturally sweet – once more detoxification is the only way.

For women, the vagina

In puberty, girls can find that they begin to have a vaginal discharge which usually precedes the onset of menstruation. Research has shown that in cultures where clean, natural diets are eaten, vaginal elimination, especially periods, has been scanty, lasting for as little as a day without any accompanying suffering. The fact that fragrant pantyliners and 'ultra'-absorbent sanitary towels are available for sale in the West strongly suggests that something is not quite right with our experiences of these natural house-cleaning processes. The heavier the menstrual flow and the stronger the odour, again, the more we are in need of addressing our internal condition.

Our own experiences and those of other women following a more raw diet have proved to us beyond the shadow of a doubt that diet has a huge part to play in how these eliminations affect us. Some of us used to suffer from quite uncomfortable PMT – for instance, feeling unusually emotional and ultra-sensitive for a few days before our periods, as well as experiencing sore breasts and bloating. However this can be completely eradicated by diet, even to the point of not knowing when the next period is due (other than by looking at the calendar)! Likewise stomach cramps while menstruating can ease considerably and even disappear with time, while the bloodflow itself can become very light, lasting between one and three days rather than the average five to seven.

Urine

The kidneys do a terrific amount of work for us, constantly keeping the blood as clean as possible by filtering out harmful substances. Many of these substances are eliminated in our urine, including excess water, salts, proteins and some acid. Those people eating a cleaner diet of largely or totally raw plant foods have discovered that their urine becomes as clear as water! This is a reflection of the cleanliness of the blood. During detoxification, however, it will become darker and stronger-smelling than usual, so this is a good time to drink more water in order to assist the process and dilute the wastes.

Anus

Although it's the last port of call here, often the first sign of rapid elimination for you will be via the rear exit! Whether through diarrhoea or due to a general ongoing change in your toilet habits, you can bet that the body is going to use this most obvious elimination channel as often as possible. As uncomfortable or awkward as it may appear at first, be assured that the symptoms will soon pass. Of course, if diarrhoea persists for a time which concerns you (such as a few days) you may wish to consult your doctor or naturopath, but usually it will clear up quickly and leave you feeling all the better for it. It is very important to keep hydrated when suffering from diarrhoea, so drink plenty of water.

Other symptoms during detoxification can be less obvious and not necessarily physical in nature. You may find that you begin to experience strange emotions, feel a little more sensitive than usual, or may feel excessively irritated without apparent reason. The whole spectrum of emotions can be experienced along the way, so be prepared! The reason for this is quite simple – the state of your body affects the way you think and feel quite significantly. Imagine your river again and visualise how, when fresh clean water is poured into a slightly murky stream, all the rubbish comes rushing up to the surface to be cleared. This bodily cleansing process is identical – there's displacement going on and naturally it causes quite a stir!

The good news is that, whatever your experience of detoxification, it will not last for ever. Not only that, but it probably won't last as long as you think. With each passing phase, the symptoms get fewer, and with each cycle you begin to feel better than you have done for years.

How long does the cleansing last?

This obviously depends on how much you need to clean out of your system. On average, there is usually a period of about one month (but for some, up to six months or so) of quite noticeable symptoms, such as rashes, headaches, stomach upsets and so on, although these are far from being an everyday occurrence and in between you will feel great. This dwindles down to occasional clean-outs that can erupt seemingly out of the blue, but are usually over in a day or two. These can sometimes seem like a severe cold or an attack of flu, and yet never last long and usually leave you feeling even more alive. Also those of us who live in the Western world are rarely able to live in a completely pollution-free area or to eat a complete diet of organic foods, these occasional cleanses (maybe once or twice a year, and less for some) will persist throughout our lives because we will always have some inner debris to cleanse out.

As an added bonus, due to a 'cleaner', healthier body, your immune system becomes that much stronger and any infections or illnesses that do occur are generally very mild and are over very quickly.

Hiccups along the way

Addiction strikes back!

So there you are, happily incorporating more and more fresh, raw foods into your daily diet and feeling great, when suddenly you hear an insistent inner voice demanding chocolate. As you have been merely incorporating more raw food into your diet instead of forcing yourself to cut out the so-called 'naughty' foods, there should be no panic involved. If part of you wants chocolate, then why not?

However, it's useful to be aware of which part of you this desire is coming from. Sometimes such behaviour can be purely emotion-based, a kind of rebellion against yourself or the new approach. If you decide to have the chocolate – and you more than likely will in the early days – then don't let guilt spoil your enjoyment but do carefully observe how you feel afterwards. You may decide from then on that chocolate will be your one 'treat', but quite soon you may not like how your body reacts after eating it, and it might seem like more of a treat not to have it. Only time will tell.

Bingeing – the final fling

It is not unusual for people to go on complete food 'frenzies' when they've been 'good' for some time! This can be really unsettling as you wonder what has gone wrong and yet it is a very common stage that most people go through. One day, after weeks of including more fresh salads, luscious fruits and all manner of other new goodies in your diet, and gradually letting go of more junky foods, the aspiring intuitive eater says: 'Well, this is all very nice *but...*' and goes right back (and often in a more extreme way) to their old ways of eating. Suddenly sweets, cakes, biscuits, crisps, ice cream, chips, cheese, bread, quiches, cold baked beans, chocolate, even things which haven't been eaten since childhood – almost anything can come back on to the scene.

As predictable as this is, and even somewhat enjoyable at the time, the net result is equally predictable: the person will usually emerge from the binge feeling sick (very sick indeed mostly), often a little sad, slightly dumbfounded and generally completely exhausted by the experience. Although an extreme example, this is actually very similar to the way your body used to feel inside every day.

Sometimes yo-yo-ing in this way can go on for a while

and it doesn't feel like fun any more. Indeed, if it becomes a regular habit, it can be extremely uncomfortable for some people, not just physically but mentally and emotionally too. If this happens, especially if you have a history of eating disorders or preoccupation with food, it is the easiest thing in the world to feel a whole range of negative emotions about yourself, as if you've somehow 'failed'. The vital first step is to let go of the guilt. There are organisations available to help those with severe eating disorders (see Useful Contacts); however, for most people experiences like these are a natural occurrence that disappear with time, not a sign of an eating disorder. The next time this happens to you, allow yourself to fully experience it – good and bad – and trust that this alone will make bingeing happen less and less. As drastic as it may sound, the truth is that what we are experiencing at such times is the evidence of just how much of a hold cooked and processed foods have over us.

For many years I was a compulsive eater who thought about food constantly. This meant that I relentlessly struggled with my weight and suffered from long periods of depression. Finally, I decided to eat as close to a 100 per cent raw food diet as possible. Since then I have lost nearly three stone in weight, only think about food to plan meals and look forward positively to every day.

John Robinson, UK

Cravings – a real need, an emotional fix, or a detox experience?

Cravings are similar to addictions except that their hold or pull is somewhat weaker and more sporadic, and not necessarily for something we would eat every day – things like toast and peanut butter or a Chinese takeaway, for example. At this stage the reasons for cravings are likely to be twofold rather than threefold as before – either it's something working its way out of your system (ie it's in your bloodstream waiting to be expelled, therefore spurring the craving) or it has an emotional memory attached to it, something you are keen to recreate. If you are now eating a wide range of raw foods it is extremely unlikely that your craving is a search for a nutrient (that's just wishful thinking!), as everything you need for a healthy and vibrantly alive body can be found in natural, raw, unprocessed organic plant foods.

If your reasons have emotional origins (like finding a particular food comforting or reminding you of happy times), now is a great time to once again practise the self-observation exercises described in Chapter 3 to discover if the foods really do comfort you or make you feel happier, and also to see if you can put up with any of the accompanying side-effects, such as feeling bloated. This alone might provide you with adequate inspiration to turn around some of these 'unhelpful' uses of food and to find more positive ways to satisfy these needs. Instead of trying to recreate past feelings with food, why not choose a more positive activity like having a nurturing warm bath, getting stuck into a good book or meeting up with friends?

Breaking through – the return of clarity

I'm very new to raw foods – one month. I've noticed a difference in my energy levels and disappearance of cravings. I feel great.

Linda Bechard, USA

Succumbing to addictions, cravings and bingeing may not be the most enjoyable of experiences in the short term, but they are most definitely invaluable in the long term. By incorporating more simple foods you are giving yourself much more of an opportunity to cleanse than before and it can sometimes seem like too much all at once. By giving in to one of these cravings or addictions you therefore slow the process down, and although it may feel like a failure it can often be the best possible thing to do. First, it gives you a great opportunity to learn more about your various selves, to skip the guilt and apply compassion instead. Second, it can act as a reminder of how good you feel on raw natural foods, with the benefits becoming more and more obvious as time goes by. Just watch in amazement as your commitment comes on in leaps and bounds!

Rescue remedies

Stomach pain, indigestion, bloating, wind

In the early days especially, it is quite common to experiment or binge and get less than great results. When experimenting, if we're talking raw organic plant foods, the problem is not the food itself but the way it has been consumed. Whether you've eaten too much for emotional, social or habitual reasons or have just eaten a poor combination, the best fix is firstly to STOP! Then make a cup or two of peppermint tea (peppermint is tremendously useful in alleviating digestive problems and relieving pain) and avoid eating again until a strong appetite returns.

When it does return, be very gentle with yourself and eat just one food, perhaps a juicy fruit, or a very simple light meal. Let your senses direct you to whatever feels appropriate and you'll be feeling back to normal in no time at all.

Teeth sensitivity

This mostly occurs when people overeat on sweet fruits such as grapes, dates or dried fruits, or those high in acids such as pineapple and some citrus fruits, and consequently any weaknesses in the gums or teeth are irritated. If caught early enough this can simply act as a learning experience as long as the fruits are laid off for a day or two. More pronounced sensitivity is likely to be a sign that the emphasis needs to be shifted away from the fruit in question for some time, or at least reduced significantly. Instead, begin to introduce more green foods (such as lettuce, kale, spinach, watercress etc) to restore mineral balance and fatty foods to complement them (such as soaked nuts, seeds and avocado) and the problem should be relieved. Make sure you continue to brush well and floss regularly to catch any stray fibres, and consult your dentist to see if your sensitivity could be rectified by treatment.

Feeling unbalanced

Perhaps you've overeaten on fruit and feel all 'sugared-out' or you've overeaten on nuts and feel rather clogged up. Again, take the lesson and feel happy that you have reached the stage where you are actually hearing and/or feeling your body's responses to your eating habits – not so very long ago you may not have known your body even had a response!

The food-combining chart in the Appendix spells out which foods go best with which. The great thing is that each time you experiment with your diet you will be learning another lesson about the way your body works and reacts. The more raw food you eat, the stronger the feedback will be and you'll be building a relationship with your body that you may never previously have dreamt possible.

I have been 100 per cent raw for only seven weeks but the changes have been astonishing. My sense of taste has changed completely. My sense of smell has become so much more acute. My excrement and sweat are virtually odourless. My saliva tastes wonderful. I have this wonderful light feeling and my eyesight has improved. After exercise my recovery rate is so much quicker ... no more eczema in my ears, my prostate – which had been enlarged – has shrunk and I have no more torn muscles from pushing myself too hard in the gym. If you are thinking of going raw, just get on and do it!

Bruce Hunter, UK

Clearing out more than just your body

Mental and emotional detoxing

At first you may think nothing of it, or maybe not even realise you're doing it, but the chances are that as you begin detoxifying physically, you will also start 'dejunking' your mind. It could be anything from getting some long overdue paperwork out of the way or making some phone calls to friends that you have been meaning to do for a while, to thinking about redecorating your living space or clearing the attic.

With physical detoxifying you know what is going on – a displacement of old for new – and here the process is actually much the same. You may find it less and less comfortable to have excess 'stuff' on your mind and want to get rid of it or deal with it as soon as possible. Even if it only expresses itself as spring-cleaning one room in a mad, inspired flurry, this could well be the outward sign of a mental detox.

Before long you'll start getting far more done, with increased efficiency. As you body begins to clean itself out, your inner vitality level rises considerably – so your thoughts begin to change, your emotions become more balanced or audible to you and your general awareness becomes heightened. It is as if you are beginning to function on another level.

During the weeks and months that follow, you will

be more than pleasantly surprised at the changes you begin to see in yourself. For example, in the early days many people often remark on how light and calm they now feel, while others, previously plagued by mood-swings or depression, are excited by their new-found *joie de vivre*. Others still have even described vivid dreams of flying and waking up feeling incredulous at the memory of how free and alive they felt!

This can be a very exciting time as it becomes apparent – perhaps for the first time in many years – that you are beginning to experience aspects of your true potential that you had no idea existed before. Therefore discovering, developing and living a high-energy lifestyle is clearly an attractive option. Knowing how to incorporate this new way of eating into your current lifestyle, and learning how to maintain it, naturally becomes the next area for consideration.

Why raw? Because it made perfect sense to me. What did I discover? In a nutshell(!) – a dramatic rejuvenation of both my looks and health, increased energy levels, clearer thoughts, a more positive outlook and a 'high' no drug could ever give me. Now there's no turning back!

Laura Skorupa, UK

5 Living in the Real World

Your food choices often affect those around you, and this in turn affects yourself once more. In this chapter we offer some suggestions as to how you can easily and successfully integrate eating more raw foods into your everyday life whatever your circumstances. We also suggest ways of giving yourself the vital motivation and support you need to keep inspired and moving forwards, as well as ideas on how to receive help and support from others along the way.

The key to thriving in your everyday life is to do what feels most right for you at the time. Sometimes this may mean eating in a way which you would perhaps prefer not to as you juggle with your own thoughts and feelings and those of others around you, and sometimes it may be more comfortable for you to assert your preferences without inhibition.

But who knows where you will end up on your food journey? The good thing is that you don't have to know. In fact, if you're keen to learn to eat intuitively, there's actually no way you can know! So, in the meantime, let's look at some of the everyday situations you are likely to encounter along the way and how you might handle them.

Starting with you

First of all, how are you viewing this new approach in your mind's eye? Are you concerned about what others might think? Slightly embarrassed about breaking away from the pack? Nervous about explaining your dietary preferences and perhaps being thought of as fussy? Alternatively, maybe you're happy, confident and excited about making your new discoveries known to those around you? Whatever you're feeling, know that you do have a choice in that too.

Interestingly, if you look at this in depth, you could find that how you are feeling about yourself and food will often be mirrored back to you by those you come into contact with. For instance, if you are feeling a bit self-conscious, those around you could well start to ask lots of (what feel like) probing questions, picking up on your insecurities and thus making you feel more self-conscious still! However, you can use this as an exercise to find out just where your insecurities lie – the more confident and happy you are about what you're doing, the easier and more enjoyable the whole experience will be. This may not stop the questions but their focus could change so that instead they take the form of admiring comments and enquiries about what you're doing.

Relationships

There are no two ways about it, if your partner is also keen to enjoy the same kind of health and vitality as you, it will be much easier and more enjoyable than going it alone. But, if your partner is nonchalant or even concerned about your changes, what then?

Well, nonchalance can be quite easy to deal with. If both partners fully respect each other's differing lifestyle choices and these can coexist in the same kitchen – then fantastic. If, however, you have a partner who is not interested in what you're doing and is not concerned with their diet as it stands, their nonchalance could become rather infectious, making it very easy for you to gradually revert back to old eating patterns without caring for yourself and without inner awareness. But this isn't inevitable.

If you are unsure about compromising but still find yourself doing so, the solution is to know where your priorities lie and what feels like the right approach to take in order to maintain your sense of being acceptable and valid, even if it is different from your partner. With self-awareness and a love of the new way you are feeling, you should find that you can maintain a high raw diet very easily with a partner who is uninterested.

What about a partner who is concerned about your food changes or even against them? Maybe talking about it in a sensitive and open way will allow you the opportunity to make your feelings known, or ask her/him about their concerns and address them patiently, taking on board their opinions. At all times, try to keep the discussion balanced and sane, non-threatening and honest and...don't conduct it at the dinner table. Too many emotions, habits and traditions are caught up in food, so you're far more likely to be rational about it when you're not eating!

The key is to value yourself as an individual with a right to be unique and to make your own food choices. When this attitude matures and your self-respect increases, you may find that you also respect your partner's individuality more and you don't need – or want – to change them either.

Friends, family and colleagues

When you change your eating habits quite radically you can expect a fair number of reactions from those around you. The more people who learn about your changes, the more reactions you will get – ranging from: 'Are you sure you know what you're doing?' through to 'I wish I could do that but I just don't have the will-power'. The best thing you can do for yourself is to remain centred in your own thoughts and that way you will be confident in your opinions and how you express yourself.

If you're feeling a bit vulnerable, a quick technique for easing the pressure of the opinions of your close family and friends is to try saying something like: 'Well, it's just an experiment at the moment, but I'm really enjoying it so we'll see what happens...' Not only is it much less threatening to their sense of who you are, but also it's more than likely the absolute truth! Who knows where you're headed? When others think that it's just a phase or 'another diet', suddenly the pressure is off. While they're waiting for you to come back to your senses, you can be off exploring them!

If some people are relentless in badgering you about your dietary habits, then they obviously have some concerns of their own in the diet department. If you come across this, stay calm and collected; don't raise your guard, but instead try asking them why they have an interest in what you're eating. As long as they are not feeling attacked, you could well be giving them an arena in which to air dietary concerns that they may not get a chance to do elsewhere. You could be surprised!

Parents

Feelings and patterns of behaviour around our parents can be slightly more tricky to negotiate. Those who raised and fed you could find it very uncomfortable to see you rejecting the way they taught you to nourish yourself. They might think you are saying: 'You fed me rubbish and now I'm having to sort myself out!' Obviously no loving parent would ever consciously do anything to harm their children – they did what they felt was right with the knowledge and circumstances they had at the time.

Again, the best way forward is to try and remain balanced. When you're with them, try to make it clear in the way you communicate that there are none of those resentful feelings involved. Being light and casual about it remains the key. Perhaps you could say that you've just caught up with the latest way to eat healthily and you're having some fun with it. If it feels appropriate or if they ask, maybe try to introduce them to something you're enjoying, like a freshly squeezed juice instead of a cup of tea, or some raw triple-layer cake (see Chapter 7) instead of the usual baked apple pie. Both of these things are sure-fire winners. Most people, whatever their usual diet, ask for more of this cake, as long as you refrain from saying 'It's good for you, you'll really like it' and give them the room to relax and find out if they actually do!

If you are able to have a closer, more open conversation with them, perhaps explain why you are doing what you're doing, making it clear that this is to take care of yourself. Above all, *don't* try to change or challenge their own food ideas at this vulnerable stage – that can come later if you really feel it is appropriate.

A word to the wise!

It is not uncommon for those gradually transferring to a high raw diet to become so excited by the way they are feeling that they want to tell everyone. Due to the vibrant changes within, you may be tempted to grab even total strangers by the arm and say, 'You just *have* to do this!' Do try to resist the urge even though you may feel you have discovered gold when you first experiment with raw food! By all means answer questions and be enthusiastic if asked; but attempting to convert anyone who hasn't shown interest in your new diet is often seen as some kind of threat, or even an insult.

The truth is that many people associate their eating habits very closely with their own identity and, depending on the individual, they can take it as a criticism of them as a person. Far better to let the results speak for themselves and, when they ask you why you suddenly look so great, then let them have it! But, we repeat, do not expect, hope, assume or nag them into trying intuitive eating – you will only be disappointed. What you can do, though, is take comfort from the knowledge that you have planted a seed and it just might grow one day – maybe not tomorrow or even next year, and maybe not even in their particular garden, but because they might pass the information on to someone else who is interested.

Eating out

Eating out with a more raw diet is far from a problem. All it takes is a little ingenuity on your part and the part of the chef and it need not be any more difficult than any other meal. It may not always be as beautiful as a meal you can create yourself at home, but at least you will be eating what you really want to eat. As long as you are friendly, open and helpful about suggesting what you'd like, the staff are usually more than happy to help.

Begin by looking at the list of salads on the menu, and if there isn't one, there's bound to be a side salad at the very least. Depending on what's there, you can ask them to replace the usual eggs, tuna, dressing or whatever with an avocado or a sprinkling of nuts. If they have neither, try asking for a number of raw vegetables, such as carrot, broccoli, celery, sliced courgette, cauliflower, mushrooms and olives; if that option is not possible, how about asking them to double or treble the tomato and other salad items already there? Depending on what you have managed to successfully incorporate and the size of your appetite, you could suggest adding in some fruit like orange segments, apple slices, grapes or pineapple chunks to top it all off and give it more depth. Needless to say, you could well end up with a dish which not only delights you, but also the waiter and the chef – not to mention those you're eating with.

When it comes to eating out in some restaurants where salads are not very evident on the menu, perhaps a little more creativity is needed. If you love hot and spicy flavours, then given a bit of notice any reputable restaurant could use their ingredients to make a flaming salad, using the carrots, cabbage and exotic vegetables raw instead of cooking them.

If you don't want to invite questions from the chef about your preference for raw foods, you could always say you have a health condition which means you have to eat that way – the chances are that you won't be questioned further! In fact, some restaurants have been known to adopt new meals because of the regular requests of customers and, who knows, your favourite meal could become their bestseller in years to come. Besides, eating healthily is a growing trend – by stating your preferences you can help to make this happen sooner rather than later for the benefit of everyone, yourself included.

Dinner parties

So, you've been invited to dinner by a friend who does-n't yet know about your new approach to food. Do you mention it or do you bypass it 'this once' to avoid the hassle factor? Again, your shout. Granted, eating differently to most other people at a more intimate setting is not going to be the most appealing aspect of the evening, but there are ways round it. You could make some enquiries in advance about what was to be on the menu, then ask if any vegetarians would be attending and, if so, what they would be having instead. Depending on how the host felt about the vegetarian option, you could then go on to explain about your own choice of diet. Keep it light and humorous and say that you are more than happy to bring your own dish pre-prepared, or offer a few suggestions of what you'd like if they are keen to do the catering. As ever, it's all about communication and, besides, even though dinner parties are centred around food, people usually go for the company and the atmosphere more than anything else. If you do decide to stick to your guns when eating out, you can bet your choice will be a conversation starter if nothing else!

Weddings, birthdays and religious celebrations

Usually weddings and the like have a long lead time, so make any dietary requirements known as soon as possible and all should be straightforward. Be prepared to come up with some suggestions if necessary and try to avoid apologising – you really haven't got anything to apologise for! Who knows how many others you might encourage to have their say in the future? It seems crazy that we should compromise our real needs for fear of being different.

In fact, it was this fear of being seen as different or 'fussy' that prevented Karen from being more assertive about her real wants in social situations for four or five years. However, when she did finally make the commitment to her all raw diet, the opportunity for her to make her preferences known for the first time was at a family wedding reception. Despite her concerns about being served a boring plate of lettuce and tomato, what actually arrived was the most beautiful plate of food she had ever seen! The Maitre d' told her that the chef had been working on the concept for a whole week – it had really made him think.

Christmas and other religious festivals and customs do of course have certain foods associated with them. This is another area where you will come to your own decision about how to play things. Christmas (or similar festivals) may be the one exception which intuitive eaters make to their food needs. But after a year or two they often get to the point of not wanting to eat heavy stodgy foods any more. They want to stay wide awake to fully enjoy the whole day, rather than being slumped in a chair feeling fat and over-fed. These festivals should, after all, be a time for celebrating and enjoying life, treating ourselves and others to loving kindness. Contrary to popular belief, this does not necessarily mean with rich food, alcohol and general overindulgence that is regretted for days afterwards.

Holidays

Holidays are often seen as a great opportunity to try new foods and delicacies. Perhaps you will decide to put your new eating habits on hold while you're away, or perhaps you will go with the best of intentions and then see how it goes. Enjoy yourself, be happy and give yourself permission to do what feels best in the given situation. No one can ever do better than that.

If you are holidaying abroad and keen to stick to your eating plan it might be helpful to find out if you can take any food through customs. If so, pack yourself some packets of beans and seeds for sprouting, some nuts and dried fruit just in case they are not readily available and perhaps some dehydrated cookies, crackers and so on. Most countries will have an abundance of fresh produce from which you can make up the bulk of your diet, and more than likely you will discover some amazing new fruits and vegetables that you'll sorely miss when you return home!

If you're flying, there shouldn't be any problem on the plane itself. There are always vegetarian and vegan meals available and most airlines cater for special diets. Even fruit platters are served nowadays, but do order well in advance and it's worth double-checking at least a week before you fly. It doesn't hurt though to take fresh fruit on board the plane and eat the meal offered only if it appeals, or you can always skip eating altogether of course. In fact, you might feel all the better for it as long as you keep well watered.

Invest in yourself

Life at home

Your own home is going to become your haven as you experiment with your eating habits. You will no doubt be keen to have your kitchen complement your new lifestyle and there is definitely great scope here to make the whole experience of preparing food the most enjoyable, exciting and colourful yet.

You may not want to go as far as installing your very own juice bar – although there are some people who have – but there are certainly many ways that you can transform your kitchen to encourage your emerging intuition. This obviously depends on who else uses it too!

Of course, the process is bound to be gradual and you might start simply by bringing in a new piece of equipment like a blender or a cheap juicer and, if no one else needs them and it feels appropriate, you could remove such things as your deep-fat fryer, roasting tins or frying pans.

In Chapter 7 you can read about what the various basic pieces of recommended equipment are for and we would encourage you to invest in whatever feels right as soon as you are able. If budget is a problem, look out for second-hand equipment in local papers, health shops, magazines or through The FRESH Network. However, rest assured that eating well is absolutely not dependent on owning electrical equipment – the best processing equipment you will ever own are your teeth! Therefore everything you invest in for your kitchen will be a huge plus rather than a necessity – but life is definitely more fun for having such things around and your culinary skills will be stretched in a whole new direction.

If you're really keen to revamp your kitchen, the first thing to do is to set aside a half-day or evening in which you can take a long hard look at what you've been filling it with. If you share it with others, obviously you will have to talk your plans over with them first and maybe even assign separate cupboards to different people. Only when you know what *you* want are you free to begin the transformation.

Staying motivated

Feeling good about yourself and feeling good within yourself is a sure recipe for a more fulfilling, healthy and harmonious life. Although your eating habits will be constantly evolving in the early days, you may reach a stage where you want to commit to a more permanent intuitive high raw diet. This decision will take you beyond this book and more and more into your own experiences. When a stage as important as this is reached, it can be vital to find encouragement and support.

It can be a great help to be prepared for the lower

moments, or times of stress, when a little voice might try to tempt you back to your old ways or tell you you're crazy. The freedom factor should continue to be respected, so ideally you should always feel as if you can do whatever you want to do – even go back to your old eating habits if that is what you want. However, by this point it is quite possible that you wouldn't actually enjoy your old habitual ways anymore. If this is the case, you can help yourself immensely by having your own motivational pick-me-up plans. If life is getting you down for one reason or another and you are used to using food to cheer yourself up, be prepared for this and indulge the healthy way by having a supply of healthy sweet treats on hand such as dates, figs, raw candies and snack bars (see Chapter 7). This way you can satisfy your craving and stay on track, thus avoiding the addiction cycles.

If you are feeling generally out of sorts, remember that great health is holistic and all about nurturing yourself in each and every way – mind, body, spirit and emotions. So when you're feeling positive and full of confidence, make a list of things which you love to do, or have always been meaning to try, and then, when you are low, select something that will lift you up again – and do it!

Some people like to monitor their intuitive journey by keeping a diary of the changes that occur, so how about finding ways to chart your own? Go back to the journal in which you described your health and well-being before developing your inner awareness and see just how far you've come since then. Some people have devised charts complete with stickers and stars for their own and their family's progress and have had great fun doing so. If this kind of record-keeping works for you, then get creative!

Ongoing support and help

Doing things for yourself and maybe even by yourself is all well and good, but most of us love to socialise. As food plays such a large part in modern-day social activities, wouldn't it be good to meet other like-minded people or be able to share your lifestyle with them?

The FRESH Network (known as FRESH, for short) exists precisely for this vital role of bringing people of a like mind together. In addition it offers a wide range of books, videos, audiocassettes, kitchen equipment and other related goods to help you increase the raw food in your diet.

With the advent of more and more food scares, concerns about GMOs (genetically modified organisms), plus a surging interest in organic foods, FRESH now has more members than ever. In order to support as many people as possible, FRESH Groups have sprung up all over the UK. These groups – together with annual events, lectures and workshops – give people the opportunity to learn more, make new friends, try new foods, make bulk food purchases locally and generally just learn and explore together rather than alone. FRESH members come from all walks of life, from all age-groups, and from all over the world – but what they all have in common is an interest in a high-energy lifestyle.

Networks like FRESH exist in countries all over the world and you can find details of many of them in the Useful Contacts section at the back of this book. They are all closely networked and keep each other up to date with what's happening in their own parts of the world.

The journey out of modern-day mythology and back to the comparative safety of intuitive eating could well be one of the most transformative, exciting, fascinating and enjoyable explorations you ever make in your culinary life. Of course, for us to say it is one thing – for you to try it and know it for yourself is what will really convince you.

Raw food has changed my life. Eating cooked food I was just surviving. On raw foods I am thriving! I choose to eat raw food because I want to live my life to the fullest!
Paul Nison, USA

6 Intuitive Children

There are many reasons we, as parents, aspire to improve our children's health. No matter what reason you cite, your underlying motivation is the love you have for your child and the responsibility you feel to do what's best for them.
 Cheryl Stoycoff, author of Raw Kids: Transitioning Children to a Raw Food Diet, *USA*

A common concern for parents is: 'Yes, it may be all right for an adult to eat in this way, but what about a baby or a growing child – surely they need a conventional cooked diet?'

Of course feeding a child is an immense responsibility. But by observing the changes in yourself and by turning back to Chapter 2, you will get confirmation of just how good raw-food nutrition is and the foods that work best for adults are also best for children. The only slight difference here is that young children not only need concentrated, top-quality, easy-to-digest nutrients, but they also need less of the high fibre/cellulose vegetables (such as tough green leaves, marrows and root vegetables) although, perhaps not surprisingly, these are the ones they don't usually like anyway.

This chapter takes a practical look at dealing with intuitive eating when you have children – whether you are just planning to have a child or have a hoard of opinionated teenagers. After all, children have their own intuitive skills that can be developed – but which foods and which approaches are healthy for them? And how much should their decisions affect your own?

Pre-conception

Childhood is the crucial time for mind and body development, so naturally parents want to be able to give their young the best possible start in life.

This starts at pre–conception, as the father's and especially the mother's health are very influential to the outcome of the child's health dispositions. Genetic factors play a vital role, however: the overall health of the initial seed, the efficiency and vibrancy of the uterus and placenta, the nutrients that the baby receives to fabricate its body, plus the mother's emotional and physical well-being, all work hand in hand to determine the child's overall start in life.

Therefore the ideal is to start a more raw, intuitive way of eating well in advance of conceiving a child, so that the parents' bodies have plenty of opportunity to detox and create an optimum place in which to support eggs and grow sperm and eventually babies.

Pregnancy

During the early months of pregnancy many women experience extreme intuitive signals from their bodies in the form of 'morning sickness'. Some very interesting research has been collated by Margie Profet in her book *Protecting Your Baby-to-be*, to support the premise that standard levels of such nausea are the body's way of telling the mother to avoid certain foods. These foods, on closer inspection, contain levels of plant toxins that may be harmful to the growing embryo, and include vegetables such as onions, garlic, broccoli, mushrooms, cabbage and potatoes, as well as spices and most herbs, tea, coffee, cola drinks, barbecued and fried foods. In her book, not surprisingly, Profet concludes that the most appropriate food for the first three months, when the embryo is developing all its vital body organs, is raw fresh fruit![1]

Later on in the pregnancy, some women develop cravings, such as for hot spicy food or even bizarre items like coal. These can be interpreted in several ways, one being that often in later pregnancy women find their sense of taste diminishes and so crave more highly flavoured foods. There is also evidence that some cravings are due to a need for certain key nutrients, while others may be due to comfort-eating because of stress.

A high raw diet at any stage of this vital time will provide the mother with concentrated, easily assimilable nutrients for her own health and that of her baby. It will also help prevent the mother from gaining excess weight (a very common trait in Western countries), and so aid her flexibility, muscle tone and overall fitness in preparation for the birth and well after. However, it is also very important to take into consideration the cleansing action of raw foods and how this might affect a growing baby.

As discussed in Chapter 4, anyone relatively new to eating a high-percentage raw diet will experience some degree of detox. This is usually slow for all those taking a gentle approach to this way of being, but if you are growing a baby or breast-feeding these eliminating toxins could find their way into the developing foetus and the milk. This does not necessarily mean that it's time to get straight back to a chip and beefburger diet! Evaluate your own situation according to your overall health – the more junk food you have eaten recently, the slower you should go. A mother's body will naturally protect her unborn or breast-feeding baby, so a very gradual detoxification process should not cause any serious problems for her child. However, if your cleansing is powerful and rapid, or if you have had any powerful drugs in the past – medical or otherwise – then you should slow down the pace greatly by eating simple cooked vegetables such as stews, soups and alkalising grains such as cooked millet, along with plenty of alkalising raw leafy greens.

Naturally, food is only one factor of many to consider – exercise, emotional health, a clean environment and the need for adequate rest, are also vital to support a healthy pregnancy and birth. For advice on a joyful intuitive birth, try the Active Birth Centre (see Useful Contacts), which offers information, classes and a whole range of services for all birth scenarios.

Your new baby

On the arrival of your new baby, there are two diets to consider. Breast-feeding is now widely regarded as the best way to feed your baby, but in the West most women still only breast-feed for a very short period. The world average for weaning a child from the breast is 4.2 years,[2] yet in the UK it can be considered unconventional to breastfeed beyond 6 months. Of course all mothers and families have unique needs and circumstances and we all have to find our own best ways of dealing with them, but it's important to note that milk is almost vital to the successful growth and development of a child in its first few years. There is phenomenal information and support for longer breast-feeding, such as vital statistics and scientific backup on the advantages of human milk for the developing child, from La Leche League (see Useful Contacts).

Most families use cow's milk and yet it's so obvious

that calves have such different development and growth needs to that of a human baby. For instance, a calf might weigh about 90lb at birth and then reach about 2000lb at two years, whereas a human might weigh 8lb at birth and only reach about 20 to 30lb in two years. One of the reasons for this dramatic growth is because there is about 300 times more casein (a protein) in cow's milk than there is in human milk.[3] This is the substance that is the basis of extra strong wood glue and when dairy products are eaten, the casein coagulates forming large, dense, difficult to digest curds. We really need four stomachs like the cow to digest them. Cow's milk makes calves grow very rapidly in body structure, without the necessity of growing large or complex brains – food for thought perhaps! Basically, if cow's milk is most appropriate for a calf then surely human milk is the ideal for a baby or a child.

For those who choose not to breast-feed or are genuinely unable to, please consider the following example: if you take the milk from a nursing cow and pasteurise (boil) it before giving each feed to her calf, that young animal (in nine out of ten cases) will not survive six months. The basic process of pasteurising milk creates many unassimilable ingredients and destroys the milk's enzymes, rendering the final product a mere shadow nutritionally of what it is meant to be.[3] For instance, one of these enzymes, which specialises in breaking down phosphorus-containing compounds, is destroyed in the pasteurisation process. This makes the calcium in the milk insoluble and therefore constipating.[4]

Many find the commercial plant-based milks such as soya, oat, pea and rice milks useful for babies of six months or more, but there are far superior raw alternatives that you can make yourself – raw almond milk, for example, is a great substitute. (See Chapter 7). However, do note that these milks should not be used as a primary milk for babies as they are not sufficiently nutritionally complete.

It is important here to re-emphasise the protein issue. Most adults are taught that growing children need dairy products to provide lots of complex proteins for rapid growth. However, if we return to the biological composition of human breast milk, as touched on in Chapter 2, we will see that it is a low-protein, low-fat food which has been tailor made for baby humans! Babies and growing children do need high-quality and easy-to-assimilate proteins and fats, but not the high-density ones from the dairy farm which are specifically designed for another animal species.

For those parents concerned about raising children without animal milks, a study measuring IQ showed that children raised as vegans had equal or higher intelligence than their meat and dairy-consuming peers.[5]

Weaning

The next decision parents face is when to introduce solid foods, and which are the most appropriate. It seems that the recommended time gets earlier and earlier, and some advisers suggest eight weeks as a good time to start introducing baby food. To us this sounds suspiciously like a ploy by the baby-food manufacturers to get people to buy even more of their product! It has clearly been shown that if you introduce solid foods too soon, then your baby could be more at risk of developing allergies.[6] Also, one of the first foods that many books recommend to parents is baby-rice, which is basically a simple cooked starch – and yet babies do not develop the enzyme ptyalin (which is needed to digest such starches) in their saliva until they are at least one year old.[7] This is why some babies don't get on with bananas at first, or need them to be super-ripe so that most of the starch has been converted to fruit sugar.

Therefore we would recommend looking to your baby for advice and not necessarily strictly following the advice in child development books.

A very hungry baby does not necessarily mean that it's time to start solids. Such a baby will simply suckle more milk, which in turn stimulates the breasts to produce more – so, within a day or two, the baby is receiving more of what it is asking for. It is a sad fact, but women in our culture have been so ill informed about how their body works, particularly about the breasts and how they tailor their supply perfectly to the needs of the baby, that all too soon they give up on breast-feeding.

So what signs will your babies make when they want solid food? When it's mealtime, sit them on your lap, or very near, and they will soon get curious about what this food business is all about. At first they will just want to be able to touch food but later they'll want to copy putting it towards their faces – you needn't do anything else for them at this stage. In time they might get more successful at putting stuff in their mouth, so do make sure that what's on offer is very soft and will not choke them. At this stage, they could well only be interested in playing with food in their mouth to see how it feels and tastes, but not necessarily to eat it. Good soft foods to introduce at this point are simple mashed fruits such as pear, mango or melon. Leave the more complex soft foods like avocado and banana until later (six to nine months old) because they could result in constipation if given too early.

The important thing to stress here is to allow your baby to give you the messages – not a book. Healthy breast-fed infants will do very well on a predominantly milk diet for at least the first year and quite often will be almost two years old before they want other foods in any quantity. Obviously all children are different – some will want to eat solid foods at four months and others might take a lot longer, so don't worry. As long as babies have access to a wide range of quality foods to satisfy their appetite – are well, vibrant, curious about their environment and have a sparkle in their eye – then they are doing just fine!

As they do start to eat solids, babies are likely to want all the foods that you and your family eat, and this is when it is really important to involve them fully. Some families try to keep their baby on a very pure diet when they are not following one themselves. It doesn't work. Babies want to eat what they see you eat and, at shared mealtimes, making their food too different from the prime carer's could cause long-term problems.

For more information about specific raw foods for your baby and growing child, contact The FRESH Network.

Growing children

Given time, your child will no doubt want to experiment with food he or she sees outside the home (in shops, the media, with other people etc). It is important therefore for you to be able to allow safe experimentation and encourage self-awareness, so that your child develops his or her own intuition and confidence with food.

Most children will have a strong need to be part of their social group. From quite an early age (usually four to five years) this usually means their peers at school, their local friends or their relations. This need to 'belong' is often much stronger than that of an adult, as the child is going through unconscious inner processes of working out who they are, what they like and so on. It can manifest itself in one of two ways: either in a powerful urge to be different from, or more likely to be just like, their friends. As we already know, the marketing of processed food has become highly sophisticated in recent decades, and food advertisements are often designed to generate a high 'I want it' response from children.

But does this mean you let them eat as much junk food as they like? Well, children need to do a lot of experimenting with all areas of their lives, not just with food – especially as they enter their teens – and if they are unable to do so at home, they are bound to find other ways and places. With this in mind, do put special effort into finding good ways of keeping communication flowing with your child so that these issues can be kept in the open and, perhaps, compromises found. There's nothing worse than making food a battleground. Your child is an individual with his or her own needs, which are unique. It is worth remembering that most children will go through especially junky food phases in their teens, only to slowly replace these foods by choice as they grow older. Also, if you have given them a solid foundation of raw food in early life, then their intuition is going to be functioning in a far superior way. The bright glitzy processed foods will soon have less appeal if you allow your child to dabble.

Interestingly, you will find that by learning to trust and respect your own food responses, you will find that process of empowering your children will be much easier.

Encouraging children who are new to intuitive eating

What do you do if you have decided that intuitive eating makes sense and have started to gradually change over your own diet, but your children are cooked-food junkies and addicted to the usual rounds of pizza, bread and ice-cream? Of course it does depend a great deal on your personal circumstances: how many children you have, their ages, their diet preferences, the amount of choice they currently have, your own preferences (or otherwise) to have them change their diet, any existing health problems or tendencies and much more. There are of course many possibilities, but we'll aim to cover the basic fundamentals here.

The most important factor is that you first need to be involved in your own self-discovery process in order to show your children that you too are committed to the benefits of intuitive eating. Children are very aware of the difference between 'a nice idea' and something that their parents feel is really important. Once you are learning to value yourself more and to respect all your inner needs, your example alone will be very encouraging. You will also automatically have a wider perspective on the importance of allowing your child to develop their own self-awareness and self-esteem.

To help them do this, encourage your children to express their thoughts and feelings more fully. Of course, they may say one thing, but the need they are trying to address may be quite different. By listening in a constructive way you can help them to explore their own food intuition in whatever way works best for your family. There are now many books and organisations available to help parents learn new listening skills to improve family communication and raise confidence and develop self-esteem in both adult and child (see Useful Contacts). To create an environment of self-discovery at home might mean allowing more choice (within limits) than for yourself of the types of foods your child can eat and more flexibility around mealtimes. However, this does not necessarily mean allowing them to do anything they like. Setting boundaries on what is appropriate behaviour and food within your family is equally important, as too much responsibility too early can be unhelpful for everyone.

Yet obviously, most children are open and vulnerable to the pressures imposed by their peers and the food advertisers. Allowing them too much freedom is likely to result in children becoming addicted to the standard chips and junk food regime, so they'll need all the help and support they can get from you. However, given a wide range of 'appropriate' foods, their intuition will start working more for their benefit, naturally leading to better food choices and therefore to a happier child and a happier you.

Allowing your children to have more choice and flexibility with their food at home need not spell chaos at family mealtimes. A common concern we hear from some mothers (or the primary food preparer) is: 'But I already cook two separate meals at dinner-time because my son has food allergies and won't eat what we do. I don't want things to get even more complicated.'

You must know your own boundaries about what you are and are not prepared to do for family meals. By encouraging your child to take more responsibility for the food choices they make, you can simultaneously encourage them to prepare more of their own meals in conjunction with yours. Also, remember that the simpler the food offered, the less preparation (and washing up) needed!

A table laden with a whole range of luscious fruits and vegetables along with the chosen cooked foods makes a beautiful and enticing spectacle. You can then all gather, eat what you want from what's there, and share the special family time that comes from being around the dinner-table eating and chatting together.

The practicalities

If you want to start clearing out some of the 'unhelpful' foods from your cupboards, consult with your children about their food needs and perhaps create an area in the kitchen that is only for them – if you feel that they are old enough for such a responsibility. If not, then start changing what you give them in their day–to–day meals extremely slowly. If the changes are gradual and subtle they could well not notice, especially if you put special effort into making simpler food more enticing, through using creative presentation. For example, instead of offering just one or two types of fruit for breakfast you could start their day with a fresh fruit salad, perhaps piled high in a special glass or bowl.

If you do not want to go for the subtle 'hope they don't notice' scenario, and feel they are old enough to understand, then explain fully your actions about cleaning out the addictive, unhelpful foods from the cupboards. Show them that you are doing this because of what you have found to be the best care for your own health, and that you want to give them the best environment for their own well–being.

Raw foods can easily be jazzed up. Carrots for example can be served whole, grated, cut into very fine slithers or sticks, juiced or made into a face display with other vegetables. It's also amazing what you can do with a cucumber! Again, try tiny thin slices, very long fine sticks, flower shapes (by peeling the skin back on a chunk, exposing the core inside) or scooping out the core of soft flesh and presenting 'hula-hoops' of cucumber ready to place on fingers or stuff with dips.

This is also an excellent time to experiment more with a fruit juicer. Most children like freshly made juices and it is an extremely effective way of getting concentrated nutrients into them quickly and deliciously. You can use fruit that is in season, and therefore much cheaper, and it's a great way of using up surplus fruit that may have otherwise gone to waste. For example in the summer, when perhaps only half of a watermelon has been eaten, the other half makes a fantastic juice. Also oranges and other citrus fruits, that are perhaps slightly too sharp for young taste buds, sweeten up immensely once put through a juicer. You can also add pears or apples to carrot juice if the existing carrots are not already sweet enough.

The general rule with pre-teenagers, though, is the simpler the food the better. Obviously it depends on the type of food that they have been brought up on, but almost universally children, given the choice, will avoid the complex tastes and flavours that adults so readily seek out. So do not expect your child to want a complex salad with dressing – instead, offer them a range of the ingredients that are in your salad, but individually in separate bowls, so that they can put them together as they choose.

Getting them involved in growing foods, such as sprouts, will also help them to further develop their relationship with raw food. Keep each type of sprout separate, so that everyone can experiment to find the ones they prefer.

As with yourself, try to keep the transition to a more raw diet as gradual as possible to keep the detoxification process manageable. Typically, young children 'clean out' very quickly and with the minimum of symptoms; it's only as we get older that things can sometimes be more complicated! However, the same transitioning guidelines apply, such as keeping the child's water-level high and putting more emphasis on salads at first (see Chapter 4). Salads need not be strong green leaves if these are a problem for your child. Sweeter varieties such as iceberg and romaine are good alternatives, and salads are just as alkalising and nutritious if they consist purely of other ingredients such as cucumber, courgette, carrot and celery. Have you ever finely grated up raw beetroot or sweetcorn? Many are pleasantly surprised at the unusually sweet salad mix they make. The same goes for butternut squash and sweet potatoes which make wonderful nutty raw 'chips' if sliced very fine.

If bread plays a large part in your child's diet, and you would like this to be otherwise, start by substituting the bread for whole-wheat crackers, and then slowly change these to non-wheat ones such as rice-cakes or rye crispbreads. In time suggest alternative crackers, such as thin slices of sweet potato or cucumber, or firm leaves of lettuce. By gradually moving away from the soft slices of bread idea, the whole concept of sandwiches gradually adapts to healthier alternatives without anyone feeling that they are missing out on anything. Sandwiches are viewed as the ultimate convenience food in that you can supposedly grab a sandwich and run! However, with a bit of advance planning, if your fridge is full of 'seed' cheeses (see Chapter 7), tomatoes, cucumber and other salad ingredients that your child likes, then a quick and tasty snack can be prepared just as easily.

What if your child does not want to eat raw foods?

As mentioned before, the last thing you want on your hands is a food fight! The key here is to know what you want for yourself, your home and your child. If you are in the least bit unclear in your own intentions, then your child has, potentially, a wonderful hairline crack to exploit. For example, if you are really not sure that cutting out bread is healthy, then if you try but your child refuses, their protests could well entice you to change your mind.

The other important factor here is that a lot of parents do not make their decisions in isolation and there are often the needs of the other parent to take into account. If for instance you want to be more raw, and your partner is a pizza and cheese sandwich addict, then it is vital that you find a common stance between you about what you want for your child. This could be a compromise, but obviously food is not the only input in parenting – the love and respect between the parents and what they are able to offer the child are vital too!

So the old adage of 'know thyself' is vital here. Know what you think is reasonable for your child at their particular stage of maturity, and apply it. If your child is old enough, and it does not compromise your own needs in the house, allow some flexibility and freedom of food choices. If, however, your child is young and you want them to eat a simpler, more raw diet and you find a lot of resistance, then try the following.

Saying 'no' might be a vital way for your child to assert his/her desire to start experimenting with more independence or it may be an attempt to cause drama and conflict. If you are clear in your intentions you can try to diffuse the situation by offering a choice. For younger children, this has proved to be an amazing tool for taking the sting out of potentially flammable situations. For instance, instead of asking 'What raw food do you want this meal?', try giving a choice between two foods only. Or if your child has said 'no' to the meal choices, then offer one of the dishes in two ways, ie 'would you like your fruit salad served in a bowl, or in one of these tall glasses?' Offering choices is a wonderful way to show your child that you value their individuality and that they can make their own decisions.

Another tactic is to increase the raw content of a meal by adding more fruit and salads, without taking away any of the other foods – just as we suggested for you in Chapter 4. Raw foods need to be eaten first though. So you could make their preferred meal (eg fish and chips), but insist that they eat a bowlful of simple, sweet salad first.

If all else fails and your child will not eat anything that you offer and demands a visit to the local hamburger shop, then take a deep breath, find a way of looking after yourself and relaxing (perhaps by putting on some soothing music), and say 'no' calmly and softly. Don't let yourself get caught up in their anger. Try to remain calm and cool, allow them their shouting and whatever is needed, and move yourself out of the room if it gets too much to bear. In time they will calm down and eventually eat, as hunger will win in the end.

For some parents this might sound like a frightening prospect but it is a very important lesson for your child. They are learning from you that it's all right to have principles and stick to them, and to say no. They are also learning that it's all right for them to express anger/frustration and to let it pass, that the anger is theirs, and that adults do not need to be drawn into or swamped by another's strong feelings.

In conclusion, for optimum self-esteem and emotional and intuitive health, a child needs clear, strong boundaries on food (and all other subjects), along with a clear, gradual process of being handed more of the practical decision-making as they grow and mature.

An important final point to remember: parenting is

one of the most demanding jobs there is. Value yourself for being a 'good enough' parent, instead of berating yourself for not being able to follow an ideal. We all do our very best with the circumstances at the time – these being our own needs and state of being, those of our children, the knowledge we have and the conditions of our environment.

7 A Taste of Living Foods

I am now 'feeding' my cells. The enhanced energy and health experienced is indescribable.

Terese Kredo, UK

This chapter is where we finally get to talk serious food: what to buy, where to buy it, different ways to prepare it, and we've also included some delicious recipes to get you started.

Shopping

The best possible way to go with your food is to get it as fresh and unadulterated as possible – either by growing your own or buying from a local supplier who grows their own or who has freshly picked daily deliveries. Organic foods are definitely superior to commercially grown produce. Whether we're talking about vitamin and mineral content, lack of pesticides, herbicides, GMOs etc, or freshness, vitality, colour and, of course, flavour, organics win hands down. They also help to remind us about the importance of buying in season.

The only drawback with some organic food is, of course, price and availability. Currently prices are noticeably higher for organic produce although they do appear to be creeping steadily downwards and becoming more widely available too. The more of us who put our money into these foods now, the more this trend will continue.

When selecting your foods, don't forget to engage all of your senses and make shopping quite literally a multidimensional experience. Relearn how to use your nose, hands and fingers especially. By doing this you can learn to feel your way around foods to gauge how good they're going to be for you, and it soon becomes second nature to squeeze, sniff and even shake your selection, rather than simply eyeing it up.

When it comes to selecting by sight, always go for the deepest-coloured produce of the bunch. As a general rule, the darker it is the more nutrient-rich it is, so go for the darkest greens, the rubiest red of tomatoes, the deepest purple of plums. Check everything for signs of ripeness, or even decay, not just by inspecting them by eye but by gently pressing them too.

Do as the French do and sniff your fruits and vegetables. Many of us seem to have forgotten that our sense of smell is an invaluable guide as to how safe or delicious a food will be to eat. If there's no fragrance from mangoes and other tropical fruits you can bet that they won't be very delicious to eat either. When it comes to coconuts, give them a good shake to make sure that their milk is swishing around inside – if it isn't, you can assume it's too dried up to be palatable. And finally, don't forget to use your newly awakened sixth sense and allow yourself to stray from the shopping list and be drawn to ingredients you may never have tried before. By using all your other five senses, as well as your intuition, you can begin to 'tune into' foods and be guided by your body – a much more satisfying and exciting way to shop.

Supermarkets

Many of us, owing to time and convenience, buy our food from the local supermarket. In previous years this has meant quite a limited supply in terms of top-quality produce, as their organic range only seemed to include potatoes and carrots. Thankfully things have begun to change, with a wider range of organic fruits and vegetables appearing every year. Shopping at supermarkets does raise many ethical and environmental concerns, however, so again you must do what feels right for you.

As alternatives, or to complement your supermarket shop, do try health food shops and wholefood warehouses; farmers' markets; pick-your-own and farm shops; mail order companies; and organic box schemes. Local grocers, standard markets and Asian or oriental shops also stock a diverse range of fruits, vegetables, nuts and dried goods – but they may not necessarily be organic.

To find the nearest health food shop or box scheme to you, try looking in the Yellow Pages, or on the Internet or contact the Soil Association. They can also tell you where your nearest farmers' market is (see Useful Contacts).

Foraging

Although it is the least commonly used resource, don't forget that many of the most nutritious foods available are growing quite literally in our own back yard. Foraging may have become a forgotten art, but it is currently being revived here in the UK and not a moment before time. Wild green leaves and herbs are incredibly nutritious and what many of us may think of as weeds, actually provide a whole assortment of foods. You can find such foods in gardens, woodlands, by streams and on heaths, and what's more they're totally free and as fresh as it gets. Some common examples are listed under Herbs and Wild Greens on pages 167–8, plus some more edible wild plants under the fungi section on page 177. Be sure to correctly identify the foods you collect, though, and only forage in places free of domestic animal wastes and other pollutants such as car exhausts and industrial discharges.

What foods are best?

To become in touch with your natural instincts the best thing you can possibly do, as we have seen, is to eat as much fresh raw plant food as you can. Second, make as much of that plant food organic as possible and, third, keep meals as simple as possible. This way your body will only have a few very high-quality foods to deal with at a time, so the feedback you get will be much stronger and clearer. 'Mono eating' is the term applied to eating just one food per meal and this is incredibly useful for getting really in touch with your body. However, especially at first, you'll be keen to investigate the bright new world of raw-food recipes, and we'll come to this later in the chapter. It is fascinating to discover just how many different types of produce there are to be explored. Just take a look at the lists that follow – if you thought eating raw foods was going to be limiting, think again!

Fresh fruits

Fresh fruits are the most delicious of all foods and can be complete meals in themselves. Scientists and nutritionists the world over agree that fresh raw fruits are not just beneficial to health but support vibrant and superior health. As investigated earlier, we are frugivorous by design so fruit is the perfect food for humans. It is also extremely cleansing. When selecting, go for fruit that is as ripe as possible. Many imported fruits have been picked underripe, are often frozen or kept at too low temperatures, sometimes irradiated, and of course – if not organic – heavily sprayed and treated. As always, go organic wherever possible or find local fruit trees to forage from.

The following have all been bought in the UK, although obviously not always in the standard high street grocers! Those listed with an asterisk(*) indicate a more 'complex' fruit that takes longer to digest. For instance, some are high in fats and others have very concentrated sugars, and so on. These fruits are less ideal if you want to go on a cleansing fast as mentioned in Chapter 4.

Apple (braeburn, cox, granny smith, golden delicious, jonogold etc)
Apricot
Asian pear
Avocado *
Banana *
Bilberry
Blackberry
Blackcurrant
Blood orange
Blueberry
Breadfruit *
Cape gooseberry/Chinese lantern
Cherimoya/Custard apple
Cherry
Cloudberry
Coconut (jelly/baby coconuts are better, available from oriental shops) *
Cranberry
Date (various, most are dried or processed in some way – look out for the totally raw ones) *
Dewberry
Dragon fruit
Durian (usually imported from Thailand – expensive but worth it!) *
Fig

Gooseberry

Grape

Grapefruit (yellow, Florida, pink)

Greengage

Guava

Huckleberry

Jakfruit

Juniper berry

Kiwi fruit

Kumquat

Lemon

Lime

Loganberry

Lychee

Mango

Mangosteen

Melon (charantais, cantaloupe, honeydew, galia, crenshaw etc)

Mulberry

Nectarine

Olive (difficult to find raw unprocessed ones) *

Orange

Papaya

Passion fruit

Pawpaw

Peach

Pear

Persimmon

Physalis

Pineapple (including dwarf – the majority are picked when they are still very acid and remain that way)

Plantain *

Plum

Pomegranate

Pomelo

Quince

Rambutan

Raspberry

Redcurrant

Satsuma

Sharon fruit

Star fruit/Carambola

Strawberry

Tamarillo

Tamarind

Tangerine

Ugli fruit

Watermelon

Vegetables

Veggies are a very rich source of minerals and excellent for body-building and regeneration. After a period of eating most of your vegetables raw, the cooked variety will begin to taste very bland indeed. Let your body show you that raw veggies are the way to go and get used to chewing properly again!

Artichoke
Asparagus
Aubergine/Eggplant
Beetroot
Bok choy
Broad bean
Broccoli
Brussels sprout
Cabbage (red, white, purple, winter)
Carrot
Cauliflower
Celeriac
Celery
Chinese cabbage
Corn on the cob/Sweetcorn
Courgette/Zucchini
Fennel
Garden pea

Green bean
Haricot bean
Jerusalem artichoke
Kohlrabi
Leek
Liquorice root
Marrow
Okra
Parsnip
Potato (not ideal as these starches are very difficult for the body to break down)
Pumpkin
Radish (red, white)
Rhubarb
Runner bean
Snow pea/Mangetout
Spinach
Squash (spaghetti, acorn, butternut, pattypan etc)

Sweet potato   Yam
Turnip

Salad fruits

Bell pepper (green, red, yellow, orange)
Cucumber
Tomato (baby, beefsteak, plum, baby plum, vine etc)

Greens

Green foods are incredibly potent healing foods because they are so full of chlorophyll – otherwise known as 'liquid sunshine'. If you want to speed up detoxification, aid weight loss, chase free radicals and heavy metals from your body and generally feel supremely healthy, the more greens you can get into your diet the better – especially in the early days. Juice them, eat them in salads, even eat the larger-leaved varieties with your main courses as you would usually eat bread – whatever you have to do, just get them inside you!

Many of the herbs and wild greens can be found wild or can be grown easily yourself. Herbs have the incredible ability to completely transform a dish. Some herbs need to be avoided by pregnant or lactating women, or for those with specific health conditions. If in doubt, consult a professional herbalist or an authoritative herbal textbook.

Leafy greens

Beet greens
Chard
Chicory/Endive
Dandelion greens
Kale
Lamb's lettuce

Lettuce (cos, romaine,
little gem, flat, iceberg,
Chinese leaf etc)
Rocket
Turnip greens

Herbs and wild greens

Balm
Basil
Bay leaves
Borage
Burdock
Chamomile
Chervil
Chickweed
Chicory/Endive
Chive
Comfrey leaves
Common orache
Coriander
Dandelion
Dillweed
Garlic mustard
Horseradish
Lemongrass
Lemon verbena

Lovage
Mallow
Marjoram
Mint
Oregano
Parsley
Peppermint
Raspberry leaf
(NB Not during pregnancy
other than the last one to
three months)
Rosemary
Sage (not during pregnancy)
Salad burnet
Savory
Sea purslane
Shepherd's purse
Sorrel
Spearmint

Tarragon

Thyme

Watercress

Water mint

Wild celery

Wild garlic

Yarrow

Nuts

The use of nuts has become very distorted. Not only do many people eat them roasted and salted, which in itself is highly unhealthy (roasted nuts become toxic owing to heating their fat, and salt has many health hazards associated with it), but the fact that they are often eaten by the handful is way out of proportion with what would happen in nature. Once out of their shells nuts have a tendency to go rancid very quickly, so the guidelines for eating nuts are very different to what you might be used to.

Firstly, most nuts are usually heat-treated to de-shell them, so are therefore not raw. Cashews, for example, (which are technically a fruit) grow enclosed in a poisonous casing that has to be removed with heat in order to extract them, so even those labelled 'raw' are highly unlikely to be! With most other nuts, unfortunately, you often can't tell the difference unless you are sure of your source or try to sprout them. Even those still in their shells are often heated to preserve them. The safest bets are always going to be those you've harvested yourself, such as 'wet' walnuts or almonds (easy to remove from their shell). Try to buy your nuts whole wherever possible as any splitting or damage makes them much more likely to go rancid.

As they are so concentrated, nuts should be used sparingly, and ideally soaked before eating. This simply means putting them in a bowl of pure water for at least eight hours or overnight so that some of their enzyme activity can be revived. Not only will they taste a whole lot different, but they will also be digested much more easily. Don't soak for longer than twelve hours though and change the water after at least six hours to avoid rotting. Soaked almonds – also known as almond sprouts (although they sprout very slowly) – are absolutely sumptuous! After soaking for about eight hours or more they become really juicy and taste altogether different to their dry counterparts.

Almonds (preferably in shell, but otherwise always unblanched)
Beechmast (nut of beech tree)
Brazil nut
Cashew (technically a fruit)
Chestnut
Hazelnut/Filbert
Macadamia
Peanut (technically a legume)
Pecan
Pine nut
Pistachio
Walnut

Seeds (for eating straight)

Seeds are great for adding that extra something to salads or for incorporating into snacks. A handful of pumpkin, sesame and sunflower seeds is always welcome when you're craving heavier foods. However, as with nuts, all seeds are better for being soaked for a few hours to make them 'come alive' again, though this is more noticeable with the heavier ones than the tiny ones. Experiment and see what a difference it makes.

Aniseed

Caraway

Celery

Dill

Fennel

Fenugreek

Hemp (technically not legal to sprout/grow in some countries without a licence)

Linseed/Flaxseed

Poppy

Pumpkin

Sesame (hulled or unhulled)

Sunflower (hulled)

Wheat groats (hulled)

Small vegetable seeds (for sprouting)

These are nutritional powerhouses and taste so fresh it's incredible! Aim to eat as many freshly sprouted items in your salads and other main meals as possible. You can read more about sprouting in the next section.

Alfalfa

Brussels sprout

Cabbage

Clover

Cress	Mustard
Fenugreek	Onion
Garlic	Radish
Kale	Turnip

Greens (for growing)

Indoor greens are a fantastic way to get some extremely fresh chlorophyll-rich plants into your diet. Once you've tried sunflower 'greens' you could well be hooked!

Barley for barley grass juicing
Buckwheat (unhulled groats) for buckwheat lettuce
Pea for pea lettuce
Spelt (unhulled grains) for spelt grass juicing
Sunflower (unhulled seeds) for sunflower greens
Wheat (unhulled grains/wheatberries) for wheatgrass juicing

Beans, pulses and legumes (for sprouting)

Boiled beans look dead and lifeless and taste pretty much that way too, so no wonder the sprouting concept has become so popular! Most people are cautious about eating beans and legumes raw due to health-scares concerning the toxicity of these products when dried. Such caution is well justified. However, once you have soaked and sprouted your beans, pulses and legumes, these enzyme inhibitors and toxins are practically nullified via the germinating process and reduced to completely safe levels.

There are so many different types of beans to try to grow yourself and each one has their own distinctive taste and texture. Hummus (also spelt hummous and humous) is just one of the many delicious foods that can be made with sprouted beans.

Aduki/Adzuki

Blackeye bean

Chickpea/Garbanzo bean

Haricot bean

Lentil (brown, green, red, puy)

Lima bean

Mung bean (commonly known as bean sprouts)

Pea (green, marrowfat)

Peanut

Pinto bean

Soya

(NB Kidney beans are not listed here because they have certain toxins present that can only be eliminated through extensive cooking.)

Grains (for sprouting)

In Chapter 2 we touched on the subject of grains and discussed their relative newness to the human diet, as well as outlining why they can be a 'comforting' or 'numbing' type of food for many people. If you've been used to a high starch, bread or carbohydrate diet, a good transitional step is to sprout raw grains – you'll find them incredibly filling and a very satisfying food in the early days.

Sprouted grains are, like every other kind of sprout, far superior nutritionally than their cooked cousins. A whole variety of foods can be made from them, such as sprouted wheat bread, crackers, croquettes, crisps and wafers. They are also excellent for making raw pizza crusts and cake bases. You'll find a few sample recipes towards the end of this chapter.

Amaranth	Quinoa
Barley (hulled)	Rye
Buckwheat groats (hulled)	Spelt
Corn	Wheat
Millet	
Oats/Groats (hard to find as	
all others such as rolled,	
jumbo and porridge oats	
are heat-treated)	

Spices

Fresh or dried spices are a good way to add a certain something to foods when you're looking for that extra kick. In the early days the chances are that, after eating a highly flavoured diet, raw foods may take a bit of getting used to until your taste buds begin to awaken to their subtler flavours. In the meantime, use raw spices to jazz up foods in order to bridge the gap.

Allspice   Cumin
Anise (star of)   Mace
Aniseed   Nutmeg
Cardamom   Paprika
Cinnamon   Saffron
Clove   Turmeric

Stimulants (use sparingly)

These foods stimulate us in one way or another. Those practising serious yoga for example have long avoided garlic and onions, as they seem to enervate the body and upset inner tranquillity. However, foods like these can be very useful for giving more kick to meals or even vegetable juices, and ginger and cayenne are great for winter months when you may feel like some extra inner heat. Chillies and jalapeño peppers are other foods that may be useful when you want something stronger or hotter. Again, experiment and find out what works for you.

Cayenne pepper   Garlic (bulbs)
Chilli   Ginger
Chinese five spice   Jalapeño pepper
(cinnamon, cloves, fennel   Onion (red, white)
seed, star anise, and   Pepper (ground from
peppercorns)   peppercorns)
Curry powder (up to 20   Shallot (small onion)
spices)   Spring onion/Scallion

Dried fruits

Like nuts, many dried fruits have been heat-treated. Before even worrying about that, however, look at the packet: are they preserved with sulphur dioxide or coated in vegetable oil? If so, we'd advise against buying them, as neither will benefit you. Wherever possible, go for organic sun-dried fruits and again, as with nuts, try to soak them before eating. This will reconstitute them and make them much more palatable and juicy. If you want dried fruits you can really trust, invest in a dehydrator and make your own – see the next section for how to do this.

Apple	Mulberry
Apricot	Peach
Cherry	Pineapple
Cranberry	Prune
Currant	Raisin
Date	Redcurrant
Fig	Sultana
Mango	

Flowers

Very few people eat flowers or petals nowadays but they can be a beautiful and delicate addition to a fruit salad, main course salad, raw cake or dessert. In fact, eating flowers and blossoms can be a very refreshing experience; it can almost be like eating perfume! If flowers appeal to you, use them as often as you can to brighten up your meals and drinks. Ice cubes may not be the best choice for your teeth or digestion, but a nice touch for party drinks is to place a petal or two inside each ice cube section, pour on water and freeze. You'll end up with the most beautiful ice cubes ever. Add to a fruited water or soda (see recipes on pages 213–14) and both you and your guests will be entranced. Some supermarkets sell a mixed pack of edible flowers, but these can be hard to find. Most of those below are likely to be found in your own garden or neighbourhood. As mentioned earlier, be sure to forage in areas free of pollutants.

Borage petals	Lavender blossoms
Calendula petals	Lily petals
Chrysanthemum	Marigold petals
Citrus blossom	Nasturtium petals
Cornflower petals	Rocket flowers
Courgette blossoms	Rose petals
Dianthus petals	Sunflower petals
Dill flowers	Tulip petals
Elderflowers	Viola heads
Fuchsia petals	Violet heads
Hibiscus petals	Wild rose petals
Honeysuckle	Yucca flowers

Fungi

Mushrooms can be eaten raw or marinated in a variety of ways; they are also very cheap if you know what you're looking for and go foraging. *So make sure you're kitted out with a guidebook (or guide-person) as there are many poisonous varieties.* Fungi have a remarkable texture all of their own which makes for a great change every once in a while. There are many varieties to discover and try. One FRESH member eats them regularly with olives as a staple; another swears that they taste wonderful combined with pineapple. No doubt you will find your very own favourite combination.

Brown cap	Horse mushroom
Cep	Morel
Chanterelle	Oyster
Crimini	Portobello
Field mushroom	Reishi
Girolle	Shii-ta-ke
Horn of plenty	

Sea vegetables

Extremely rich in minerals – especially iodine – and a great salt replacement, sea vegetables are widely available through health food shops. When selecting, make sure they have been collected from clear waters rather than polluted shores. Two of the most popular are nori, which usually comes in sheets, and dulse, which comes in flakes or strips. All sea vegetables are also much better soaked first, unless they come in flakes.

Arame	Laver
Carragheen/Irish moss	Nori (green nori has been
Dulse	toasted, black has not)
Hiziki/Hijiki	Sea palm
Kelp/Kombu	Wakame

Algae

The virtues of algae products have become much more widely known in recent years. Perhaps not the most appealing of foods at first glance, the benefits to be had, especially in the early days, will probably be hard to ignore and incredibly useful. We do not usually recommend supplements as you can get more than ample easily assimilable nutrients in raw plant foods. However, these kinds of additions, which are really neither a supplement nor a true 'food' (having been dried and powdered), are the one exception. It is best to use only those certified as organic.

Chlorella
Klamath Lake blue green algae
Spirulina

Oils

Oils are another of the 'borderline' raw foods. Although very useful for making dressings and adding EFAs (essential fatty acids) into the diet, all the fats you need can be gleaned from *whole* plant foods like avocados, nuts, seeds, olives and coconuts, and even some leafy greens. Oils are technically regarded as fractured foods and therefore are not as nutritionally complete as the wholefoods from which they come. Far better to eat olives than olive oil, sunflower greens or seeds instead of sunflower oil, walnuts instead of walnut oil – whole is always going to be better. Most oils on sale have usually been heat-treated in the extraction process, so look for cold-pressed, or even better, stone-pressed oils; apparently, despite the terminology, even 'cold-pressed' doesn't necessarily mean raw.

Almond oil	Olive oil
Flaxseed oil/Linseed oil	Safflower oil
Grapeseed oil	Sesame oil
Hempseed oil	Walnut oil

Useful additions

The products listed below are store-cupboard items that you may find useful, particularly when you experiment with desserts. Remember to check labels for rawness though, especially in the case of carob, which is usually roasted.

Agar flakes (natural gelling agent made from seaweed)
Arrowroot powder (thickening agent)
Carob powder (ground from pods of the carob tree –
substitute for chocolate)
Vanilla pods
Psyllium powder (ground husks of psyllium seeds used as a
thickener)
Sea salt (although there are many alternatives such as dulse
flakes)

Buy in jars/packets

These items are available in many health food stores
and again are great ways to complement raw produce,
although many of those listed below are not technically
raw.

Almond butter **
Maple syrup *
Miso (thick paste made
from fermented soybeans,
grain and sea salt) **
Nori sheets **
Olives **

Olive paste **
Sea vegetable flakes **
Sprouted wheat bread *
Tahini (sesame seed
paste)**
Tamari (a wheat-free soy
sauce) **

*   not raw
** likely to be heat treated/pasteurised – look out for raw
    versions

Drinks

Go for water and drink when thirsty. There are differing opinions but some intuitive eaters say that the best option is to drink distilled water. This can be bought at some health food shops, but it is cheaper in the long-term to buy a small tabletop unit and distil your own – or, if you can afford it, get a purification unit installed under your sink. The second choice is to buy top-quality bottled water, in which case take a good look at the labels on the bottles and compare the sodium count (go for the lowest). Whatever you decide is best for you, whenever possible add a few drops of fresh lemon or lime juice just before you drink to add back some electrolytes. These are vital for optimum assimilation (or, as some would say, to put some life back into the water).

If you want fruit or vegetable juices, the ones on the supermarket shelves are definitely going to be pasteurised to one degree or another no matter how fresh they say they are. Those in cartons can be especially acidic and often contain extra sugar. The best way to drink your juices, therefore, is straight from the juicer so you know exactly what you're getting. You can obtain these from juice bars, some cafés, or even better (and cheaper), make them yourself. Not only are the majority of the fruits' nutrients available to you, but the water in fresh juices is also *alive*! The best water you can possibly drink.

Equipment and preparation methods

Raw food preparation is easy and fun. Some of the equipment listed below you may never have heard of, in which case you might be pleasantly surprised to find just how easy it is to transform sprouted grains into breads, sprouted beans into pâtés and bananas into ice cream.

Don't worry if your bank balance doesn't allow you to buy the electrical gadgets you want (second-hand or new); it's amazing what you can do with a knife, chopping board, fork and bowl, and of course not forgetting your teeth.

Blending

Using a tabletop or hand blender is a great way to have fun with your food and come up with some incredible dishes with the flick of a switch. Both retail at between £20 and £30 from good electrical stores and can be used for making soups, smoothies, desserts, dressings, sauces, whips, pâtés, seed 'cheeses', hummus, nut milks, sweet treats and all sorts of other goodies. Hand blenders are usually used in conjunction with a tall container and you push down onto the food, thereby controlling exactly how much you process it. The tabletop variety can frequently be seen in cafés and even some bars for making smoothies and soups; but denser foods like pâtés, 'cheeses' and sweets need a bit more manipulating so a hand blender or Vita-Mix tabletop blender (very powerful) are the best choices here. There are pluses to both kinds of blender but the best one to buy initially is probably the hand blender, as it is slightly cheaper, easier to use (and wash up), and very portable.

Food processing

If your food processor has been gathering dust in the cupboard for years, now is the time to get it out and start experimenting. A whole range of main courses and desserts can be created with this modern whizz, and it is also great for chopping and grating vegetables if you want to prepare a lot in a short space of time. If you don't already own one, perhaps you could borrow one from a friend or buy one second-hand – you may save yourself a whole lot of money as well as giving something unused a good and valued home. If you do decide to invest in a new food processor, don't necessarily think the more expensive ones are better. Even the smallest and cheapest can probably do what you need, so read up a little before making your choice.

Juicing

A juicer is one of the best investments you can make in a living foods kitchen, and it needn't cost a lot of money. A basic centrifugal juicer can be bought from most electrical stores and can cost under £30. This is probably the best way to begin if you are new to juicing and will give you an idea of just how incredible fresh juices taste.

The general rule when juicing is to mix fruits with fruits, and vegetables with other vegetables, but not to mix the fruit and veg together. Some recipe books have begun to suggest mixing the two and while it's by no means 'wrong' it certainly doesn't make for the most digestible juice, as you will discover from mixing fruits with vegetables on your plate. The two exceptions to the rule, however, are apples and pears, which can be used to sweeten many vegetable juices that might otherwise seem unpalatable or too strong – especially 'green juices' made with dark leafy greens like kale or spinach.

There are many books now available on the subject of juicing. Some of these are general 'how to' guides, while others tell you which juices are good for which health conditions or which ones to make when you want something to perk you up, slow you down etc. The main thing is to have a go and experiment yourself to discover your own favourites – your body will soon tell you what it does and doesn't like.

Juicing is a great way to get a good clean blast of vitamins and minerals straight into your body in a very quick and easy way. There is minimum wear and tear on your digestive system because the juicing process removes the harder to breakdown cellulose (fibre) from the fruit and veg, thereby making their nutrients more easily available. The odd day or even week of only juices can be a fantastic way to spring-clean your system or speed up detoxification. If you decide to embark on such a programme, do make sure that it is at a time when you can afford to slow down, relax and – ideally – be looked after. In fact, we would strongly advise you to consult with a professional health practioner experienced in such matters or to go away for a rejuvenation retreat that specialises in juice fasting (see Useful Contacts).

Whatever juices you make and for whatever reason don't just drink your juices – eat them! Make sure you really savour them as you would a fruit you had just chewed in your mouth, allow your taste buds to really enjoy the experience rather than knocking the juice back like water. Digestion always begins in the mouth and it is vital that your body has as many signals working properly as possible – another prerequisite for eating intuitively and restoring a harmonious system.

Juicing is also the best thing to do (other than water fasting) when you have a cold or flu or are generally feeling run down. Because it requires the minimum of your body's energy to be assimilated and digested, it continues to feed you but also frees up a tremendous amount of energy for the body to direct towards self-healing and rejuvenation. Juice fasts are used at health spas all over the world and with good reason.

For those who are into regular juicing and want more

than the standard centrifugal type, there are some 'serious' juicers on the market, although they're not generally available in high street stores (see Useful Contacts). Two of the best known (and most expensive) are the Champion and the Green Power, which not only juice fruits and vegetables but can homogenise too, making them invaluable in more ways than one.

There are also manual juicers which look a little like mincers – these are quite small and simple in design and they clamp onto a kitchen work surface or table. They're operated by turning the handle while feeding in fruits or vegetables through the hole at the top. These juicers are especially useful for juicing wheatgrass and other grasses such as barley and spelt. They are ideal if you are new to such juices or do not want to invest in the bigger electric machines.

Sprouting

Sprouting beans, seeds, grains, pulses and even nuts is a growing trend and one of the easiest ways to grow your own food – you don't even need a garden. In fact, sprouts are among the most nutrient-rich foods for humans on the planet; they take the minimum of attention to grow and harvest and cost only pennies.

The 'magic' in these little treasures is in the sprouting process itself – once the legume, seed or bean begins to grow a tiny shoot, not only does the vitamin content rapidly increase, but the protein, carbohydrates and fats begin to break down to a pre-digested form. To top it all off, the enzyme content sky-rockets, making the sprouts very easy to digest.

The lists on pages 170–73 show the most commonly used foods for sprouting. Although each one may be referred to simply as 'a sprout', they all have different flavours, textures and effects on the body. Buying a simple book on sprouting is definitely a worthwhile investment in your early days as it will go into much more detail than we have space for here about what sprouts are, why they're so powerful, what nutrients they contain and how to grow them. However, you can make a start by following our basic outline.

Choose one type of seed, bean or grain (sunflower, alfalfa, chickpea and lentil are good ones to try first) and pour them into a jar until they're about an inch deep. Pour in some pure water until they are well covered (they will be absorbing this water in order to grow) and then place some mesh over the jar so they are protected from contamination but still open to the air. You can buy special sprouting jars which save you having to make your own, but a basic jam jar with any kind of small-holed mesh covering will do just as well. The soaking time itself will be different depending on which type of sprout you choose – for instance, seeds need much less time than beans because seeds have to absorb much less water in order to germinate. However, overnight is usually a good amount of time regardless of the sprout; nature does not appear to 'clock watch' as much as we do.

The next morning your soon-to-be-sprouts will have swelled up slightly and will already be looking quite different. At this point pour off the soak water and rinse them well. Make sure you drain off the rinse water as much as possible or they may begin to rot, then put them back in the jar and cover over as before. Continue to rinse each morning and evening, and within days – depending on the temperature, the amount of sunlight and the type of food you are sprouting – you will soon have your very own harvest of sprouts, all ready for eating. In order to catch them at their peak, it is best to consult a book on the subject, as the timing varies so much from sprout to sprout. However, as a rough guideline, tiny seeds and grains can be eaten within a day or two of being soaked. Grains (wheat, spelt and so on) need to be harvested quickly so that they remain sweet, otherwise they soon turn bitter. The larger beans and legumes can take up to five or six days after soaking.

With indoor greens such as wheatgrass, buckwheat 'lettuce' and sunflower greens the beginning of the process is the same, but usually after two or three days the sprouts are sprinkled onto trays of soil so that they can go on to become strong tall greens. The general rule – and again it is best to use a book specifically about sprouting – is to prepare some seedling trays an inch deep with good quality earth or compost and then scatter the sprouting seeds or grains over the surface. There is no need to bury them or cover them – in fact it's better not to, they will take care of that themselves.

Make sure the sprouts are reasonably distributed over the soil so that they're neither too crowded nor too sparse, give them a quick watering and cover with black plastic or some kind of lid for three days. After this time, take off the covering and place the tray on a light windowsill and you should see that they have taken root and are beginning to grow. They will be a rather strange yellow or brownish colour at this stage as they have yet to make their chlorophyll – this will come now that they are out in the light. Continue to water every day as much as the soil dictates and within a week or two you will have trays of indoor greens ready for harvesting. You can harvest them simply by snipping the greens as close to the bottom as possible with a pair of scissors or a sharp knife. Simple, straightforward and absolutely scrumptious!

If you have never grown your own sprouts or greens before, you are likely to be rather in awe of the whole process as you watch them transform from an unassuming and probably brown-looking embryo to a fully fledged sprout or green. It is like witnessing a miracle day by day and is, of course, wonderful for children to watch.

Dehydrating

Dehydrators are not yet well known in the UK, but can help to provide an invaluable source of dried or crunchy foods when you're looking for something to get your teeth into.

In a living foods kitchen dehydrators take the place of the cooker. They operate at very low temperatures (usually less than 48°C), thus drying out the foods rather than killing them. This ensures that the enzyme content of foods is retained as well as most of the vitamins and minerals. Rather than transforming the food biochemically like a cooker would, all they do is eliminate most or all of the water, thus making foods either more concentrated, crunchy or chewy, or preserving them for later use.

Dehydrators can be used in a variety of ways and, as they operate on low temperatures, are very economical to run, even though they are in operation for twelve hours or more at a time. You can find some sample recipes on pages 204–205, but here's a brief list to give you some idea of the diverse range of foods you can create: dried fruits such as apple rings, banana chips and peach slices; dried vegetables such as onion rings, tomato rings and cucumber or courgette chips; herb sprinkles and seasonings; bread replacements such as wheat crisps, grain crackers and seed wafers, and a delicious range of sweet treats such as fudge, fruity chews, cookies and biscuits. We think the dehydrator's time has come!

water on a sheet of nori seaweed, and prepare to create the best alternative sandwich you've ever tasted.

There are no rules here – you can add in chopped veggies, salad fruits, spreads, dips, sprouts, greens, herbs, nuts, seeds – whatever you can fit basically!

Fill the leaf or sheet with a satisfying line of your chosen combination and then just roll up. Leave a little room at the ends, though, or you could find yourself with half the filling spurting out!

Candies and sweets

Sweet treats are ideal for children (young and old!), parties, journeys, after-dinner treats, snacks or just whenever you want that sweet something but don't want to reach for chocolate. One FRESH member found that by making a large batch and storing them in the fridge, whenever a craving struck he would go for these and avoid the junkier options.

Sweet treats can be as simple as a handful of raisins, or a combination of any of the following: dates, dried figs, raisins, sultanas, dried apricots, sesame seeds, sunflower seeds, crushed or whole nuts, sprouted wheatberries, raw carob, shredded coconut, tahini, vanilla, cinnamon, nutmeg, aniseed, poppy seeds.

Below are some very basic recipes to get you started. If you're mixing by hand or blender rather than using a food processor, you may wish to add some water or a little fruit juice to the mixture. Some taste better if refrigerated for an hour or two before serving and all keep for a few days – although they might not last that long! For something quick and easy, which is sweet and savoury all at once, try the simple but classic medjool date stuffed with a single almond or hazelnut.

Sesame snowballs

Mix: 1 cup of tahini, half a cup of chopped dates, 2 tablespoons of raw carob powder, 4 tablespoons of sesame seeds. Shape into balls and roll in shredded coconut.

Simply fudge

Mix: 1 cup of tahini, 1 cup of raisins, half a cup of grated coconut, 4 tablespoons of raw carob powder, half a teaspoon of vanilla. Shape into balls or squares.

Sprouted wheat balls

Mix: 1 cup of sprouted wheat (two days old), quarter of a cup of chopped nuts, quarter of a cup of seeds, 1 cup of raisins (soaked for two hours). Shape into balls and if desired roll in coconut.

Cakes and pies

If you thought cakes were off the menu you can stop worrying! Raw cakes are bursting with life and taste incredible. Here are two to get you started, but there's plenty more where they came from!

Raw apple pie

For the crust blend: 2–3 cups of soaked or fresh dates, 1 cup of walnuts or almonds ground to flour, three-quarters cup of shredded coconut (optional).

For the filling mix: 4 grated apples, 4 apples blended, 1 cup of soaked raisins, juice of one lemon, 1 tablespoon of cinnamon.

Sharon's triple-layer raw food cake

An ultra-rich-taste sensation – wonderful as a birthday cake or dinner-party centrepiece. Prepare in a glass dish with fairly deep sides.

First layer: Crush enough almonds to cover the base of a dish to a depth of 2cm, add some soaked dates to the mixture so it binds the nuts together and spread across the dish to make the base.

Second layer: Mash 3 or 4 ripe bananas, add in a handful of chopped dates, a handful of shredded coconut, and some exquisite tropical or seasonal fruit (strawberry, mango, papaya are good ones). Mix well together and pour on to almond base about 4cm thick. Smooth over.

Third layer: Mix some tahini with carob powder to a medium dark brown colour – make enough to cover the top of the cake in a quite fine layer. Smooth on as best you can – it's a bit tricky at first.

Decorate with seasonal fruit – kiwis are good, as are

strawberries, raspberries, blackberries, or sprinkle with coconut.

Ice creams

We described how to make basic ice cream in the freezing section on page 191. The two central methods are blending fresh fruits and freezing in a tub/ice cream maker or feeding frozen fruits through a homogeniser.

For basic ice cream, banana is always the best option. Then add in other fruits, fresh or frozen, depending on which method you're using and what effect you're after. If you want a smooth ice cream, blend or homogenise all the ingredients together. If you're after something that little bit different, consider adding in chunks of fresh or dried fruit or chopped nuts at a later stage to create a 'tutti-frutti' effect.

Ideas for added extras: crushed nuts, carob powder, sesame seeds, soaked or dried fruits, small cubes of fresh fruit, some seeds or spices, flowers to decorate. Soaked raisins sprinkled over the top are fantastic!

Ice creams are also wonderful added into, or as an aside to, raw pies and cakes, especially if you've used a date and almond base/crust.

In all cases: if blending, use *fresh* fruits then freeze; if homogenising through a juicer, use *frozen* and eat immediately.

For a topping: If blending – blend fresh fruits with a tiny amount of water or juice to make a sauce.

If homogenising – push through *fresh* fruits to make a purée.

Mangoberry bliss

Blend/homogenise: 2 bananas, 2 mangoes, 2–3 tablespoons of any berries.

Tutti-frutti

Blend/homogenise: 2 bananas. Then mix in: chopped cherries, raisins, finely chopped apple or pineapple.

Tropical sunset

Blend/homogenise: 2 bananas, 2 large chunks of pineapple.

Strawberry seduction

Blend/homogenise: 2 bananas, a handful of strawberries.

Choco dream

Blend/homogenise: 2 bananas, raw carob to taste.

Coco-nutty crunch

Blend/homogenise: 2 bananas. Mix in: a sprinkling of coconut and 5 or 6 soaked, peeled, then chopped almonds.

Juices

Their reputation goes before them and their taste and effects say it all – juices are absolutely delicious and they give you an instant feel-good buzz. If your appetite for breakfast lessens, or as an alternative to your usual cuppa, try starting the day, or precede your evening meal, with a fruit, vegetable or green juice.

Fruit juices are the easiest of all and you can use one or more fruits to come up with some fantastic straight juices or combinations. Vegetable juices are slightly more of an art form, so invest in a juicing book to give you some ideas. Green drinks are very potent, incredibly healing, and speed up detoxification. Wheatgrass juice is one such example. For larger drinks (wheatgrass can only be taken in very small measures), leafy greens such as kale and spinach are used with maybe some sprouts and apple to sweeten.

Drink your juices as soon as they are made – even before you have washed the juicer. That way you'll get optimum nutrition and the greatest benefits.

Smoothies

If you want something thick and creamy just like a milk shake, smoothies are the answer. Not only are they filling and delicious, but they are devoid of all the cream and sugar that the usual fast food equivalents contain.

As with raw ice cream, banana is the usual base for a smoothie owing to its thick and creamy qualities. Blend one large banana or two small ones, add the rest of your chosen ingredients and then add water until the desired consistency is reached. Smoothies can make great toppings for fruit salads and mueslis as well as being snacks in and of themselves. For the ultimate indulgence, make your smoothies as usual, and then add some raw ice cream.

The best recipes are often the simplest ones. Try adding just one or two fruits. Pineapple, peach, nectarine, orange, date, guava, mango, kiwi, papaya and berries are among some of the best. Sesame and almond are also good subtle additions, as are vanilla and carob powder.

Nut, grain and seed milks

Almond milk is the classic among raw milks. It's really just as simple as blending soaked almonds up with some water, but it tastes far better if the almonds are sprouted and peeled first, with the resulting 'milk' strained through a fine muslin or tea strainer.

Other good milks to try are: cashew, sesame, sunflower, hemp, coconut. Grains are good too, but more of an acquired taste than the nuts which most people adore. All are great sweetened up with some fresh or dried fruits, such as dates or apricots, or with a little added carob powder for a chocolatey flavour.

Flavoured waters and sodas

Plain water tastes perfectly good to a clean palate, but if you're looking for a little bit of flavour without the food value of juices or smoothies, why not try making your own flavoured waters? It can be as simple as squeezing some lemon, lime or orange juice into your glass, or adding a dash of vanilla, or you can stir in some crushed berries pressed through a tea strainer or a small amount of some other fruit juice. A good way to do this quickly and easily is to freeze some excess fresh juice into an ice cube tray so that you have a ready supply, and then simply drop a cube or two into your glass.

Fizzy water is not the ideal drink for the human body as it introduces unwanted carbon dioxide into the bloodstream. Commercial carbonated drinks are actually one of the most acidic foodstuffs you can ingest, and they do a great deal of damage to the body. Many stories abound about human teeth being completely dissolved when left in a glass of fizzy cola, and what's more they're true.

As most fizzy waters have been artificially carbonated, the best one to go for is Perrier, which is naturally sparkling. Some Perriers come with added flavourings already, but it is much better to make your own. Again, choose a fruit juice that tickles your taste buds – for example, if you add grape juice you've got an incredibly healthy and delicious wine replacement. Go one step further and add a scoop of ice cream to your chosen tipple and you have a magnificent fizzy float.

These are just for starters – let your creativity go crazy! For details of how to gain access to further recipes and whole menu suggestions, see the Reading List.

After seventeen years on a raw food regimen, I really do not think about it much. I just eat what I love, as everyone else does. The difference is that my food loves me back; providing me with optimum health, a sense of living ethically and a clarity of mind that few have ever experienced.

Dr Douglas Graham, athletics coach, Florida, USA

raw food combining chart

POOR

PROTEINS
nuts (most), seeds,
grain cereals and beans,
soybeans, peanuts, olives, sprouts
(mung, lentils, alfalfa, radishes)

STARCHES & FATS
grain sprouts, corn,
whole grain cereals, dry beans,
peas & peanuts, potatoes, oils,
winter squash, carrots, beets

GOOD **GOOD**

VEGETABLES
leafy greens, buckwheat lettuce, wild greens,
radish greens, asparagus, sunflower greens,
cabbages, cucumbers, bell peppers, watercress,
broccoli, green beans, celery

POOR TO FAIR

POOR **POOR**

SUB-ACID FRUITS
apples, apricots, sweet
cherries, fresh figs, mangoes,
papayas, pears, peaches,
sweet plums, grapes

FAIR **POOR**

FAIR **FAIR**

ACID FRUITS
grapefruits, lemons, limes, oranges,
pineapples, pomegranates,
sour plums, tomatoes, strawberries

SWEET FRUITS
bananas, dates, figs,
persimmons, raisins,
dried fruits: apples, figs, prunes

POOR

IMPORTANT NOTES
Avocados are best combined with acid or sub-acid fruits or green vegetables.
All melons should be eaten alone.
Do not mix more than four foods from any one classification. At one meal do not mix food from more than two classifications.
Eat fruit by itself on an empty stomach. Let 20 to 30 minutes elapse after eating fruit and before eating other foods.
Three hours should elapse after eating other foods before eating fruit again.
EACH GROUP ONLY CONTAINS A SELECTION OF THE FOODS AVAILABLE

Notes

1 Introduction – What is Intuitive Eating

1. McCance and Widdowson, 'Composition of Foods', MAFF Reports, 1946 and 1991

2 The Inside Story

1. Dr T De la Torre, *Psycho-Psysiopathy*, vol. 3, Imprento Tormo, San José, 1957
2. Norman W Walker, *Colon Health: The Key to a Vibrant Life*, Norwalk Press, Prescott, AZ, 1979, p4
3. Information published by the Colonic International Association, Tring
4. Paul Kouchakoff, *The Influence of Food Cooking on the Blood Formula of Man*, Proceedings of the First International Congress of Microbiology, Paris, 1930

5. Harvey and Marilyn Diamond, *Fit for Life*, Bantam, London, 1987, p26

6. Ibid., p48

7. Humbart Santillo, *Intuitive Eating*, Hohm Press, Prescott, AZ, 1993, p84

8. Dr Joel Robbins, *Health Through Nutrition*, Audiocassette 1

9. Dr Douglas N Graham, *Nutrition and Athletic Performance*, Marathon, FL 1999, p20

10. Ibid., p23

11. Ibid., p32

12. Ibid., p19

13. Ibid., p49

14. Dr Max Gerson, *A Cancer Therapy*, Totality Books, Del Mar, CA, 1958, p80

15. Graham op. cit., p47

16. Santillo op. cit., p76

17. Ibid., p80

18. Dr Edward Howell, *Enzyme Nutrition*, Avery Publishing, Wayne, NJ, 1985, pp5, 70

19. Robbins, op. cit.

20. Francis Pottenger, *Pottenger's Cats: A Study in Nutrition*, Price-Pottenger Foundation, La Mesa, CA, 1983

21. Robbins, op. cit.

22. C Zioudrou, R Streaty and W Klee, 'Opioid Peptides Derived from Food Proteins: The Exorphins', *Journal of Biological Chemistry* 254:2448S9 (1979)

23. Ann Wigmore, *Be Your Own Doctor*, Avery Publishing, Wayne, NJ, 1982, p8

6 Intuitive Children

1. Margie Profet, *Protecting Your Baby-to-be*, Little, Brown, Boston, 1995
2. R Lawrence, *Breastfeeding: A Guide for the Medical Profession*, Mosby, St Louis, MO, 1988, p246
3. Harvey and Marilyn Diamond, *Fit for Life II: Living Health*, Bantam, London, 1987, p245
4. Harvey and Marilyn Diamond, *Fit for Life*, Bantam, London, 1987, p107
5. KW Shillam, et al., 'The Effect of Heat Treatment on the Nutritive Value of Milk for the Young Calf: The Effect of Ultra-High Temperature Treatment and of Pasteurisation', *British Medical Journal* 14, (10 November 1960), 403
6. Susannah and Leslie Kenton, *The New Raw Energy*, Vermilion, London, 1995, p39
7. FR Ellis, et al., 'Veganism, Clinical Findings and Investigations', *American Journal of Clinical Nutrition* 23:3 (1970), 249
8. 'Baby Shouldn't Be Rushed to Eat Solids', *Los Angeles Times*, 13 September 1984
9. *Fit for Life II: Living Health*, p293

Recommended Reading

There are many excellent publications available on the all-round health benefits of raw foods. Listed below are just a few of the books we and many others have found useful.

Those marked * are imported specially by The FRESH Network and sold by mail order. The remainder can be found in all good bookshops but are also available through FRESH's mail order department. Call or write for their free catalogue.

* Abramowski, Dr OLM, *Fruit Can Heal You!*, Custodian Publishing, Fremont, CA, 1981
* Alexander, Joe, *Blatant Raw Foodist Propaganda*, Blue Dolphin Publishing, Nevada City, 1990
Cairney, Edward, *The Sprouter's Handbook*, Argyll Publishing, Argyll, 1997

* Clement, Brian R, with Theresa Foy DiGeronimo, *Living Foods for Optimum Health*, Prima Publishing, Rocklin, CA, 1998

Diamond, Harvey and Marilyn, *Fit for Life*, Bantam, London, 1987

Diamond, Harvey and Marilyn, *Fit for Life II: Living Health*, Bantam, London, 1987

* Graham, Dr Douglas N, *Nutrition and Athletic Performance*, Marathon, FL, 1999

* Howell, Dr Edward, *Enzyme Nutrition*, Avery Publishing, Wayne, NJ, 1985

Kenton, Susannah and Leslie, *The New Raw Energy*, Vermilion, London, 1995

* Kulvinskas, Viktoras, *Love Your Body*, 21st Century Publications, Fairfield, Iowa, 1972

* Santillo, Humbart, *Intuitive Eating*, Hohm Press, Prescott, AZ, 1993

* Shannon, Nomi, *The Raw Gourmet*, Alive Books, Burnaby, BC, 1999

* Stoycoff, Cheryl, *Raw Kids: Transitioning Children to a Raw Food Diet*, Living Spirit Press, Stockton, CA, 2000

* Wigmore, Ann, *The Hippocrates Diet and Health Program*, Avery Publishing, Wayne, NJ, 1983

* Wolfe, David, *The Sunfood Diet Success System*, Maul Brothers Publishing, San Diego, 1999

Useful Contacts

UK Organisations

The FRESH Network
P.O. Box 71
Ely
Cambridgeshire
CB7 4GU
Tel: 0870 800 7070 (national rate)
Fax: 0870 800 7071
e-mail: info@fresh-network.com
www.fresh-network.com

A comprehensive support and information service on all aspects of raw food diets. The Network exists to help people, no matter what diet they follow, as they do not endorse or recommend only one way of eating. FRESH offers a yearly membership (including magazines and newsletters), an extensive mail order service (including books, videos, juicers and other equipment) and holds regular seminars, workshops and socials throughout the year. Call or write with an SAE for a free enquiry pack.

The Vegetarian Society
Parkdale
Dunham Road
Altrincham
Cheshire
WA14 4QG
Tel: 0161 925 2000
Fax: 0161 926 9182
e-mail: info@vegsoc.org
www.vegsoc.org

The Vegan Society
Donald Watson House
7 Battle Road
St Leonards-on-Sea
East Sussex
TN37 7AA
Tel: 01424 427393
Fax: 01424 717064
e-mail: info@vegansociety.com
www.vegansociety.com

British Natural Hygiene Society
Shalimar
3 Harold Grove
Frinton-on-Sea
Essex
CO13 9BD
Tel: 01255 672823

Other useful organisations (UK)

Organic food

The Soil Association
Bristol House
40–56 Victoria Street
Bristol BS1 6BY
Tel: 0117 929 0661
Fax: 0117 925 2504
e-mail: info@soilassociation.org
www.soilassociation.org

The Soil Association offers a wide range of services including advice on how to find your nearest supplier of organic produce.

Friends of the Earth
Campaign for Real Food
26–28 Underwood Street
London N1 7JQ

Tel: 020 7490 1555
Fax: 020 7490 0881
e-mail: info@foe.co.uk
www.foe.co.uk

Greenpeace
True Food Campaign
Canonbury Villas
London N1 2PN
Tel: 020 7865 8100
Fax: 020 7865 8200
e-mail: info@uk.greenpeace.org
www.truefood.org

Miscellaneous organisations (UK)

Eating Disorders Association
1st Floor
Wensum House
103 Prince of Wales Road
Norwich NR1 1DW
Tel: 01603 621414
Youth helpline: 01603 765050
Fax: 01603 765050
e-mail: eda@netcom.co.uk
www.gurney.org.uk/eda/

The Colonic International Association
16 Drummond Ride
Tring
Hertfordshire
HP23 5DE

Send SAE for full listing of practitioners of colonic hydrotherapy within the UK.

The British Society for Mercury Free Dentistry
221 Old Brompton Road
London
SW5 0EA
Tel: 020 7370 3132
Fax: 020 7244 0286
www.mercuryfree.co.uk

Send large SAE for full listing of dentists practising without mercury within the UK.

Parenting organisations (UK)

Creative Parenting Fellowship
P.O. Box 14
Carmarthen
SA33 5YH
Tel: 07000 270230

Founded by Helena Eastwood, they offer courses and support on parenting and communication skills.

Parent Network
2 Winchester House
11 Cranmer Road
London SW9 6EJ
Tel: 020 7735 4596
Parent enquiry line: 020 7735 1214
Fax: 020 7735 4692
e-mail: info@parentnetwork.demon.co.uk

Courses and support on parenting and communication skills.

Active Birth Centre
25 Bickerton Road
London N19 5JT
Tel : 020 7482 5554
Fax : 020 7267 9683
e-mail: info@activebirthcentre.com
www.activebirthcentre.com

Range of courses, support and merchandise to prepare families for childbirth and beyond.

La Leche League
P.O. Box 29
West Bridgford
Nottingham NG2 7NP
Tel: 020 7242 1278
www.stargate.co.uk/lllgb

Information, courses, support and merchandise to prepare families for childbirth and beyond.

Practitioners/teachers (UK)

Elaine Bruce
Elaine Bruce Living Foods
Holmleigh
Gravel Hill
Ludlow SY8 1QS
Tel: 01584 875308
Fax: 01584 875778
www.livingfoods.co.uk

Elaine is a qualified naturopath; she was trained by Dr Ann Wigmore and runs courses on all aspects of living foods.

Prof. Rozalind Gruben AHSI RSA
Health Unlimited
1 Cassidy Place
New Town Road
Storrington
West Sussex
RH20 4EY
Tel/Fax: 01903 746572
e-mail: rozgruben@aol.com

Professor Gruben is an international lecturer and health and fitness educator. She offers personal health consultations with an emphasis on fitness and raw vegan nutrition according to the philosophy of natural hygiene.

Karen Knowler
c/o The FRESH Network
P.O. Box 71
Ely
Cambridgeshire
CB7 4GU
Tel: 0870 800 7070
Fax: 0870 800 7071
e-mail: karen@fresh-network.com

One-to-one consultations available on all aspects of intuitive eating, especially dealing with the practical and emotional aspects of transitioning to a raw food diet.

Keki Sidhwa ND, DO
British Natural Hygiene Society
Shalimar
3 Harold Grove
Frinton-on-Sea
Essex
CO13 9BD
Tel: 01255 672823

Dr Sidhwa is editor and publisher of *The Hygienist* magazine and founder of the British Natural Hygiene Society. He has fasted over 25,000 people during his time as a naturopath. Consultations in London available.

Jill Swyers
Tel: 020 8870 7041
Fax: 020 8870 6706

Jill is a certified living foods health educator, as awarded by the Hippocrates Health Institute, USA. She has over thirty years of catering experience and teaches groups how to prepare sumptuous living foods menus. Private catering by arrangement. Personal one-to-one consultations also available.

Mail order (UK)

Most foods mentioned in this book should be easily available through a good health food store, or found growing wild local to you.

Seeds for sprouting, wheatgrass etc.

The Organic Gardening Catalogue (Chase Organics)
Tel: 01932 253666
Fax: 01932 252777
e-mail: chaseorg@aol.com

Mail order supplier of seeds and gardening equipment. Excellent supply of sunflower, buckwheat and wheatberries for growing indoor greens.

Greenseed Company
Tel: 020 8789 7897

Trays of top-quality wheatgrass by mail order, delivered overnight ready for juicing.

Fertile Fibre
Tel: 01584 781575

Mail order supplier of organic coir compost (from coconut trees) useful for growing indoor greens, wheatgrass etc.

Other foods

Clearspring Direct
Tel: 020 8746 0152
e-mail: mailorder@clearspring.co.uk
www.clearspring.co.uk

Mail order supplier of sea vegetables.

Suffolk Herbs
Tel: 01376 572456

Mail order supplier of organic herbs.

Equipment

All equipment mentioned in this book (juicers, dehydrators, sprouting equipment etc) is available through The FRESH Network (see page 222). Call 0870 800 7070 for their free mail order catalogue.

International support

The following organisations all publish a regular newsletter/magazine and offer support and help services.

Living Nutrition
P.O. Box 256
Sebastopol
CA 95473
USA
Tel: 707 887 9132
e-mail: dave@livingnutrition.com
www.livingnutrition.com

Also offers help and advice on healing colitis and Crohn's disease through the use of a raw-food diet.

Nature's First Law
P.O. Box 900202
San Diego
CA 92190
USA
Tel: 619 229 8259
e-mail: nature@rawfood.com
www.rawfood.com

The Fruitarian Network
P.O. Box 293
Trinity Beach
Queensland 4879
Australia
Tel/Fax: 07 4057 7273
e-mail: fruitnet@ozemail.com.au
www.islandnet.com/~arton/fruitnet.html

Justa Bananer
Lundavägen 62
232 52 Åkarp
Sweden
e-mail: tyling@algonet.se
www.algonet.se/~tyling/justaeng.htm

Boletin Crudivegano
Lista de Correos
29100 Coin
Malaga
Spain
Tel: 608 489 975

Naturlich Leben
Bund Fur Gesundheit
Talstr, 36
D-52525 Heinsberg
Germany

Tel: 02452 22678
Fax: 02452 101078
e-mail: bfgev@t-online.de

European retreats/healing centres

Ázoe Health School
C/Juan Fernandez
43 4B
30204 Cartagena (Murcia)
Spain
Tel: 629 46 11 44

Ázoe practise sustainable permaculture and teach 'The Mucusless Diet Healing System' as written by Prof. Arnold Ehret.

Moinhos Velhos
Cotifo
8600 Lagos
Portugal
Tel: 351 82 687 147
Fax: 351 82 687 697
e-mail: t00070@mail.telepac.pt
www.moinhos-velhos.com

Juice fasting programme with alternative therapies and yoga.

International retreats/healing centres

Ann Wigmore Foundation
P.O. Box 399
San Fidel
NM 87049
USA
Tel: 505 552 0595

Retreat and healing centre based on the living foods programme as taught by Dr Ann Wigmore.

Ann Wigmore Institute
P.O. Box 429
Rincon
Puerto Rico 00677-0429
USA
Tel: 787 868 6307
Fax: 787 868 2430
e-mail: wigmore@coqui.net
www.annwigmore.com

Retreat and healing centre based on the living foods programme as taught by Dr Ann Wigmore.

Creative Health Institute
918 Union City Road
Union City
MI 49094
USA

Tel: 517 278 6260
Fax: 510 278 5837
e-mail: creative@creativealternatives.org
www.creativealternatives.org

One to three week cleansing and detoxification programmes offered.

Hippocrates Health Institute
1443 Palmdale Court
West Palm Beach
FL 33411
USA
Tel: 407 471 8876
Fax: 561 471 9464
e-mail: hippocrates@worldnet.att.net
www.hippocratesinst.com

Founded by Dr Ann Wigmore and Viktoras Kulvinskas, MS, now directed by Brian Clement. A comprehensive rejuvenation programme for those seriously ill or looking to learn the whole living foods programme firsthand.

Optimum Health Institute – Austin, Texas
Route 1
Box 339-J Cedar Lane
Cedar Creek
TX 78612
USA

Tel: 512 303 4817
Fax: 512 332 0106
E-mail: russnees@optimumhealth.org
www.optimumhealth.org

One, two, three and four week detoxification
programmes available.

Optimum Health Institute – San Diego
6970 Central Avenue
Lemon Grove
CA 91945
USA
Tel: 619 464 3346
Fax: 619 589 4098
e-mail: optimum@optimumhealth.org
www.optimumhealth.org

One, two, three and four week detoxification
programmes available.

Tanglewood Wellness Center
5825 Tanglewood Drive
Bethesda
MD 20817
USA
Tel: 301 320 9299
e-mail: lorenlock@aol.com
www.vibrant-living.com

Supervised fasting retreats, vibrant living seminars and raw food preparation classes. Run by international health lecturer Loren Lockman.

Rest of Your Life Health Retreat
P.O. Box 102
Barksdale
TX 78828
USA
Tel: 830 234 3488
Fax: 830 234 3599
e-mail: vvvhaag@swtexas.net
www.naturalhygeine.intent.net

Supervised fasting, juicing or monotropic diet plans.

The Tree of Life Rejuvenation Center
P.O. Box 1080
Patagonia
AZ 85624
USA
Tel: 520 394 2520
Fax: 520 394 2099
e-mail: healing@treeofliferejuvenation.com
www.treeofliferejuvenation.com

Rejuvenation centre run by Dr Gabriel Cousens.

Index

acid-forming foods, 40, 44, 60, 197
addiction, 6, 60, 69, 70, 93, 111, 113, 115, 133, 149
adenoids, 21
ageing, 50, 52, 61
alcohol, 40, 59, 70, 71, 76, 130
algae, 178
alkaline-producing foods, 40, 140–1, 153
allergies, 65, 66, 70, 150
almond butter, 180
amino acids, 49
amphetamine, 60
animal products, 45
anorexia, 14
anus (elimination system), 109
anxiety and fatigue, 4, 83
appetite, 20, 37, 116, 127, 146
apple rings, 190

appropriation, 36, 37
arrowroot powder, 180
arthritis/joint inflammations, 46, 57
Asian shops, 161
assimilation, 7, 32, 36, 37, 51, 69
autointoxication, 35
avocado, fruity soup, 201
awakening plan/process, 10, 11, 28 see also intuition
Ayurveda, 36
Ázoe Health School, 234

babies/babyhood, 19
  allergies, 144
  first solids, 144–6
backsliding, 9
bacon, 21, 24
baked foods, 52, 98
banana chips, 190

banana ice cream, 191–2 *see also* ice cream
beans, pulses, legumes, 54, 56, 131, 171–2, 182, 186, 187, 188
    baked beans, 21, 112
    bean salads, 194
beef, 40, 45
bingeing, 5, 74, 112–3, 115
biscuits, 21, 112, 190
blender/blending, 182–3
bloating/wind *see* stomach pain, flatulence
blood pressure, 45
blood sugar/sugar levels, 39, 48, 49 *see also* diabetes, hypoglycaemia, insulin
bloodstream (for elimination), 104–5
body building, 74, 165 *see also* calorie questions, skinny, weight loss industry
body shape, 13, 100
Body Shop, The, 105
boiled foods, 52
Boletin Crudivegano, 233
bowel movement, 35, 101 *see also* anus, constipation, elimination
    bowel cancer, 35
    irritable bowels, 66
bread, 38, 47, 60, 76, 78, 79, 112, 148, 153, 172, 182, 194
    bread substitutes, 204
    home-made, 16
    pitta bread, 99
    toast, 60, 98, 114
    wheat bread, 173, 180, 204

white, 21, 24, 48
    with/without butter, 23
    wholemeal, 24
breastfeeding, 20, 140, 141–2, 144–5
    weaning, 144–5
British Natural Hygiene Society, 224
British Society for Mercury Free Dentistry, The, 226
Bruce, Elaine, 228
burger (meat), 8, 21, 24, 140, 156, 194
    lentil burger, 203
    raw burger, preparation, 202
butter, 21, 26

carob powder, 180, 191, 192, 196
caffeine, 59
cakes and pies, 112, 194, 208–10
    baked apple pie, 125
    raw apple pie, 209
    raw triple-layered cake, 125, 209–10
calcium, 67, 69, 143
calories, 4, 19
    calorie books, 15
    calorie burning capacity, of body, 46
calorie counters/counting, 74, 82
cancer, 35, 56, 61
    carcinogenic, 46
candidiasis, 65
canned foods, 52
carbohydrates, 38, 41, 47, 51, 172, 187

cardiovascular disease, 45
cereal crops/products, 47, 59, 60
cheese/processed cheese, 12, 13, 21, 22, 26, 67, 112, 154, 194 *see also* seed cheese
chemical fertilizers, 2
chicken, 40
childbirth, 19
children's health, 137
chips, 4, 8, 19, 21, 22, 25, 82, 91, 112, 140, 149, 156 veggie chips and crisps, 205
chocolate, 4, 8, 16, 22, 68, 71, 75, 76, 82, 93, 94, 111, 112, 207
cholesterol, 47
chronic ailments, 3, 45, 56 chronic fatigue syndrome, 65
cigarettes, 76
cleansing *see* detoxification, elimination
Clearspring Direct, 231
cocaine, 60
cod, 24
cod liver oil, 57
coffee, 40, 52, 71, 76, 98, 139 *see also* caffeine
cola drinks, 139
cold/flu, 2, 20, 102, 103, 104, 106, 110, 185 *see also* nose
coleslaw, 24
Colonic International Association, The, 226
comfort food/comfort eating, 60, 74, 76, 81, 139
concentrated foods (low water content), 97

constipation, 34, 143, 145
consumerism, 64
convenience foods, 15, 22, 154 *see also* junk food
cookies, 22, 131, 190, 194
cooking/cooked food, 7, 18, 35, 36, 41, 43, 49, 52, 53, 55, 57, 58, 59, 70, 93, 94, 103, 113, 136, 148, 150 *see also* baked foods, boiled foods, fried foods, grilled foods, processed food, roasted foods
courgette chips, 190
cow's milk, 20, 141–2 casein, 142
crackers, 131, 153, 173, 194, 196, 205
cravings, for food, 4, 8, 9, 48, 69, 70, 81, 93, 97, 113–5, 134, 139, 207
Creative Health Institute, 235–6
Creative Parenting Fellowship, 226
crisps, 21, 22, 112, 173, 205
croquettes, 173
crudités, 205
cucumber chips, 190, 202

dairy foods/products, 16, 20, 40, 41, 45, 79, 142, 191, 192
De la Torre, Dr T, 30, 217 *n* 1
degenerative diseases, 6
dehydrate/dehydrators/ dehydrated food, 190–91, 193
depression/mood-swings, 113, 119

dessert, 175, 182, 193, 194, 195
detoxification (also detox), 96–7, 101–10, 113, 139, 140, 153, 166, 185, 236, 237 *see also* toxic elements
  mental and emotional, 118, 139
symptoms of, 102,
diabetes, 48
Diamond, Harvey and Marilyn, 218 *n* 5, 219 *n* 3, 219 *n* 4
diarrhoea, 109 *see also* elimination
digestion/digestive processes, 32, 34, 37, 38, 41, 47, 51, 176, 185, 195
digestive organs/system/juices/enzymes, 7, 34, 35, 38, 51, 58, 104-5, 107, 184
diet, 11, 15, 16, 19, 25, 26, 27, 30, 32, 44, 49, 60, 62, 64, 69, 94, 103–4, 108, 112, 122, 124, 125, 131
  and health, 26
  diet-related illnesses, 8, 56
  diet study, 57
  dietary life, 12
  dieting programmes, 4
  modification, 81
  special diet, 131
  standard Western/British, 34, 79
dips and spreads, 194, 195, 202, 205–6, 207 *see also* guacamole, hummus, salsa
dizziness, 103

dopaminergic, 60
dressings, 152, 182, 194, 198–9 *see also* salads
drinks, 181, 194
  distilled water, 181
  fruit, vegetable juices, 181, 194, 211–2
drugs, 34, 40, 60, 66, 76, 119, 140

ear infection, 102
eating habits, 4, 22, 34, 79, 80, 95, 117, 123, 126, 131, 132, 133
  changing of, 4–5
  disorders, 75, 113
  Eating Disorders Association, 225
eating out, 10, 127–8, 129
eczema, 20, 61, 117
eggs, 13, 26, 127
elimination cycle/process/organs, 25, 32, 35, 36, 46, 104–9 *see also* bowel cancer, constipation, detoxification
Ellis, FR, 219 *n* 7
emotional eating, 75–6
emotional expression, 75–6, 87, 88
energy levels/consumption, 6, 9, 28, 59, 65, 77, 100, 104, 115, 119, 158, 185
environment, harming and caring for, 63, 160
enzymes, 41, 51, 53
  enzyme-depleted/-empty diet, 51, 52

essential fatty acids (EFA), 45, 46, 47, 179
eyes, state of, 100, 117
  impaired vision, 46
  short and long-sightedness, 57
eyes and ears (as elimination organs), 105–6

facial bone structure, 58
fast food, 6
fat/fats, 19, 43, 44–7, 48, 69, 74, 130, 143, 187, 191
  bad fats, 44
  cooked fats, 44
  EFA, 45
  fatty acids, 47
  good fats, 44
  in salads, 198–9
fatty/sugary foods, 4, 21, 41, 116
  high-fat diet, 20
  low-fat diet/foods, 22
  low-fat rule, 23
Fertile Fibre, 231
fibrous foods, 48, 137–8
  breakdown of fibres, 184
fish, 12, 21, 38, 40, 41, 67, 156
fizzy drinks, 21
flatulence, 38
flowers, as food, 175–6, 204, 210
food allergies, 65, 150
food growing, 152, 171
  sprouting/sprouts, 54, 70, 152, 168, 169, 170, 171, 172, 173, 182, 186–9, 207, 230–1

food obsessions, 74, 91
food processor, 183
food sharing, 71
foraging, 161–2, 163, 176, 177
freezing, freezers, 191–2
FRESH Network, The, 17, 132, 135, 136, 146, 177, 207, 220, 222–3, 232
fried foods, 23, 52, 139
Friends of the Earth, 224–5
fruit, 25, 32, 37, 38, 40, 41, 43, 49, 56, 63, 98, 99, 112, 117, 131, 139, 150, 159, 161, 194, 195, 199
  citrus, 116, 152
  dishes, 194, 195–6
  dried, 55, 116, 131, 175
  frugivorous, 162
  fruit sugars, 47
  fruitarian, 32
  fruited drinks, 176
  fresh fruit, list of, 162–4
  fresh juices, 53, 98, 125, 152, 184, 192, 212
  fruity chews, 190
  heavier, 97
  lighter, 97
  seasonal, 209
  tropical, 63, 160
Fruitarian Network, The, 233
fudge, 190
  simply fudge, 208
fungi, 161, 177 *see also* mushroom

gender stereotyping, 76
genetically modified organisms (GMOs), 135, 159

genuine hunger, 6
Gerson, Dr Max, 218 *n* 14
glucose, 43
gout, 50
grains/sprouted grains, 38, 41,
    47, 54, 60, 172–3, 182, 187,
    188, 202, 203, 204, 205
    grain crackers, 190, 202
grain drugs, 59–61
grain milks, 194, 213 *see also*
    cereals
Graham, Dr Douglas N, 218 *n*
    9–13, 15
gravy, 194, 199, 202
greens/leafy greens, 38, 46,
    54, 55, 138, 141, 153, 161,
    166–8, 207, 212
    for growing, 171, 189
    green energy soup, 200
    green drinks/juices, 184,
    194, 212
    indoor greens, 188
Green Seed Company, 231
Greenpeace, 225
grilled foods, 23
Gruben, Prof. Rozalind, 228–9
guacamole, 202, 203, 204,
    206
guilt about eating, 9, 82

hair, strengthening of, 100
hair loss, 46
ham/ham salad, 22, 24
headaches, 2, 36, 61, 65, 97,
    103, 105, 110
Health Through Nutrition,
    218 *n* 8
healthy foods/diet, 24, 25, 68

health food shops, 47, 160,
    177, 180
heart diseases, 50, 56, 57
hemp oil, 46
herbs and spices, 38, 55, 139,
    161, 205, 207 *see also*
    spices
    herbs and wild greens,
    167–8
    flavouring seed cheeses,
    201–2
herby tomato soup, 200
heroin, 60
Hippocrates Health Institute,
    61, 236
homeostasis, 39
holistic approach, to
    food/holism, 5, 9, 62
holistic health, 15, 60, 134
hot dog, 21
Howell, Dr Edward, 52, 218, n
    18
hummus (also hummous,
    humous), 172, 182, 203,
    203, 205
hyperactive/-activity, 20
hypoglycaemia, 48

ice cream, 8, 16, 21, 112, 148,
    182, 191–2, 194, 196,
    210–11
    banana, 191–2
    choco dream, 211
    coco-nutty crunch, 211
    mangoberry bliss, 211
    strawberry seduction, 211
    tropical sunset, 211
    tutti-frutti, 211

ice cubes, 176
iodine, 177
immune system, 35, 36, 111
'inappropriate' foods, 81, 103
infection, 57, 58, 111
insulin, 48
intensive farming, 2
intuition, 8, 11, 27, 28, 59, 66, 68, 80, 81, 82, 132, 160
   awakening of, 9
   children and, 10, 146, 150
   intuitive abilities, 83, 84
   intuitive eating/eaters/diet, 5, 6-7, 12, 63, 69, 79, 95, 99, 112, 120, 126, 130, 133, 136, 138, 148, 181, 185, 229

juice/juicing/juicers, 183–6, 211–2, 214
   juice fasting, 185, 234
junk food, 5, 15, 93, 100, 112, 140, 147, 149, 207
Justa Bananer, 233

Kenton, Leslie and Susannah, 26, 219 n 6
kidney troubles, 46
   kidney stones, 50
   urine, 108–9
kinaesthetics, 88
Knowler, Karen, 229
Kouchakoff, Paul, 36, 217 n 4

La Leche League, 141, 227
lasagne, 194
Lawrence, R, 219 n 2
lettuce, 99, 116, 202
light food, 17

linseed/flax oil, 46
liver and kidney problems, 46
living foods, 27, 54, 194
   living water, 53
Living Nutrition, 232
Lockman, Loren, 238
lollipops, fruit, 191

magnesium, 69
malabsorption, 34
marinades, 194
maple syrup, 180
margarine, 45
mayonnaise, 26
   garlic and herb mayo, 206
McCance and Widdowson, 217 n 1
meat, 21, 24, 38, 41, 44, 49, 57, 78–9, 143
   meat-based diet, 32
   meat products, 59
   packaged meat, 12
   red meats, 40
   white meats, 40
medication, 40
   medication problems, 34
   on medication, 40
meditation/contemplation, 16, 84, 89
meningitis, 57
menstruation/periods, 107–8
   PMT, 108
   stomach cramps, 108
metabolic processes, 43
microwaved foods/ microwaving, 52, 54
milk, 22, 26, 57
   milk shake, 21

minerals, 44, 51, 53, 59, 69, 116, 158, 177 *see also* sea vegetables

miscarriage, 46

miso, 180

Moinhos Velhos, 234

mono eating, 162

monosodium glutamate, 16

molecularly altered foods *see* cooked food

morphine, 60

mouth (eliminative organ), 106–7

mucoid plaque, 34

muesli, 24, 60, 194, 196–7 ingredients and toppings, 197, 213

raw muesli, 197

muscle tear, 117

mushroom, 127, 139, 177 *see also* fungi mushroom soup, 200

nails, 100

natural living/natural foods/ natural diet, 15, 25, 35, 41, 62

Nature's First Law, 232

Naturlich Leben, 233–4

nervous system problems, 57

neutral foods, 38

nightmares, 103

nose (elimination organ), 106

nutrition, 12, 15, 41, 42, 43, 48, 54, 62 nutritional advice, 17 nutritional properties of food, 1–2, 4

nutritional requirements, 80

nutritional research, 15

optimum nutrition, 35

nuts, 32, 38, 47, 53, 54, 55, 116, 117, 131, 161, 168–9, 207 cashew casing, 168

list of, 169

milk, 182, 194, 196, 213

soaked nuts/sprouting, 168, 169, 186

obsessive behaviour, 6

oils, 47, 179 *see also* EFAs, nuts, plant food, leafy greens extraction processes, 179

old age/elderly people, 3 *see also* ageing

olives, 46, 127, 180 olive cream, 206 olive paste, 180, 204

onion rings, 190

opioid, 60

optimum foods/nutrition, 9, 61

Optimim Health Institute- Austin, Texas, 236–7 San Diego, 237

organic foods, 15, 29, 99, 111, 135, 158–9, 160, 162, 178, 224–5 organic box schemes, 161 organic farmers' market, 63 organic plant food, 114, 115 sundried fruits, 175

Organic Gardening Catalogue, The, 230

osteoporosis, 50
overcooking/undercooking, 192
overeating/overfed, 81, 130

palm kernel oil, 46
paralysis, 57
Parent Network, 227
parenting organisations, 226–7
pasta, 47, 48, 60
pasteurised foods, 52
patés, 182, 193, 194, 195, 201, 203, 204, 205
peanut butter, 114
peppermint tea, 116
pesticides/herbicides, 2, 158, 159 *see also* GMOs, organic foods
pH level (acid/alkali balance), 39
phosphorus, 69
pizza, 21, 60, 92, 93, 148, 154, 194,
    creating toppings, 203–4
    making own pizza, 202–4
plant foods, 26, 30, 32, 52, 108, 162, 178
    plant-based milks, 143
pollution, 34, 63, 110
pork, 40, 45
potatoes, 21, 38, 47, 49, 160
    baked potatoes, 24, 98
    jacket potato, 25
Pottenger, Francis, Jr, 57, 218 n 20
power foods, 26
practitioners/teachers, 228–30

pregnancy/childbirth/ babyhood, 19
    Active Birth Centre, 141, 227
    and raw diet, 139–41
    foods to avoid, 139, 166, 167
    intuitive birth, 141
    morning sickness, 19, 139
    pre-conception phase, 138–9
processed food, 7, 16, 20, 21, 36, 41, 43, 56, 59, 70, 99, 147–8
    processed cat food, 58
Profet, Margie, 139, 219 n 1
prostate, 117
Protecting Your Baby-to-be, 139, 219 n 1
proteins, 13, 38, 43, 49–51, 72, 143, 186, 201
    high protein diet, 44, 50
    protein-deficiency, 67, 69
Psycho-Psysiopathy, 30, 217 n 1
psychological conditioning, 72
psyllium powder, 180
puberty, 22
puddings, 194

quiche, 25, 112

raw foods/nutrition (also simple foods), 7, 8, 16, 17, 18, 19, 26, 28, 36, 38, 40, 41, 46, 51, 52, 53, 55, 57, 63, 64, 65, 79, 91, 92, 93, 94, 95, 96, 97, 99, 100, 108, 111, 113, 114, 115, 117, 119, 123, 127, 136, 215

and pregnancy, 138–41
cake/cake base, 173, 175
candies, 134, 193, 194,
    207–8
children and, 137–57
in everyday life, 120
introducing in diet, 98–9
milks *see* grains, nuts, seeds
pizza crust, 173
preparation and equipment,
    182–92
Raw Energy, 26
shopping for, 158–61
transition to, 153, 229
real food desires, 80, 91
recipes, 2, 92, 192–3
    raw recipes, 11, 162
    recipe books, 11, 184
relaxation, 89, 97, 185
reproductive system, disorders
    of, 58
Rest of Your Life Health
    Retreat, 238
retardation, 46
retreats/healing centres,
    234–8
rheumatism, 50
rich foods, 130
rice, 21, 24, 47, 48, 60
    rice cakes, 153
    wholegrain rice, 49
roasted foods, 52
Robbins, Dr Joel, 218 *n* 8, *n*
    19, *n* 21
roll-ups, 194, 206–7
ruby rich soup, 200

safflower oil, 46

salad, 25, 98, 112, 127, 153,
    154, 155, 156, 166, 170,
    175, 194, 195, 197-8, 202
    see also dressings
    flaming salad, 128
    fruit salad, 151, 155, 175,
        192, 196, 213
    salad fruits, 166, 207
    preparation, 198
salsa, 202
    spicy salsa, 206
salt/salt replacement/no salt,
    16, 40, 177
    salt concentration (in body),
        39
    sea salt, 180, 204, 231
sandwich, 60, 68, 153–4, 192,
    194
Santillo, Humbert , 218 *n* 7, *n*
    16
seeds/seed milk, 47, 53, 54, 116,
    131, 194, 196, 205, 207, 213
    for eating straight, 170
    small vegetable seeds,
        170–71
    seed cheese, 154, 182, 201–2
    shopping by mail order,
        230–1
    sprouting, 186, 187, 188
self-awareness, 16, 67, 89, 91,
    122, 146, 149
self-empowerment, 13, 18
self-esteem, confidence, 9, 11,
    13, 73–5, 82–3, 85, 90, 149,
    156
self-observation, 82, 84,
    85–94, 114
self-reliance/-reliant, 13, 18

self-respect, 81, 82, 123
self-starvation/starvation, 14, 74
sesame, 196
    tahini sesame snowballs, 208
sex/sexuality, 14
Shillam, KW, 219 *n* 5
Sidhwa, Keki, 229–30
sinus problems, 20, 65
skin/skin tone, 100, 104, 105
    rashes, 110
    skin brushing, 105
skinny, 74 *see also* body building
sleeping disorders, 20
slim, 23
smoking, 34
smoothies, 53, 182, 194, 196, 212–3, 214
snack bar, 134, 194
soft drinks, 71
Soil Association, The, 161, 224
sore throat, 102, 103
soups, sauces, 140, 182, 194, 195, 199
    croutons, 200
    raw recipes, 200–201
spices, 173–4
sprouting/sprouts, 54, 70, 152, 168, 169, 170, 171, 172, 173, 182, 186–9, 207, 230–1
    sprouted wheat balls, 208
squashes, 21
starches, 45, 47, 48, 76, 173
stews, 52, 140
stimulants, 174 *see also* alcohol, chocolate, cigarettes, coffee, drugs, tea
stomach pain/upset/indigestion, 103, 110, 115, 116
stress, 34, 72, 75, 83, 85, 134, 139
Suffolk Herbs, 231
sugar/sugary foods, 19, 21, 47, 48, 69, 71, 76, 191, 192
    no sugar, 16
    refined sugar, 40, 45
sunflower greens, 54
Spirulina, 26
sweat glands, 107
sweet treats, 21, 48, 72, 182, 190, 194, 207–8 *see also* candies
Swyers, Jill, 230

tahini, 180
tamari, 180
Tanglewood Wellness Center, 237
tea, 40, 52, 72, 125, 139
teeth/teeth sensitivity, 58, 116–7, 133, 176, 182
teens/teenage/teenagers, 14, 20, 21, 24, 138, 147
    pre-teenagers, 152
temporary diet programmes, 4
thyroid problems, 57
tobacco, 70
tomato rings, 190, 202
toxic elements/toxins, 43, 56, 92, 105, 106, 107, 139, 140, 171, 172
Tree of Life Rejuvenation Center, 238

tuna, 24, 127
typical Western diet, 45

uncooked vegetarian diet, 62
un-cooking, art of, 192–4
urine, 108–9

vagina (as elimination organ),
  107
vaginal discharge, 107 *see also*
  menstruation
vegan/veganism, 13, 26, 65,
  131, 143
  Vegan Society, The, 213
vegetables (also veggies), 21,
  24, 38, 40, 44, 47, 49, 56,
  63, 98, 99, 131, 150, 151,
  159, 161, 165–6, 183, 199,
  205, 207
  cellulose vegetables, 138
  dried vegetables, 190
  exotic vegetables, 128
  juices, 174, 184, 212
  root vegetables, 138
  simple cooked, 140
  sea vegetables/flakes, 54,
    177–8, 180
  stuffed vegetables, 194, 195
vegetarian/vegetarianism, 13,
  24, 32, 107, 129, 131
  lacto-vegetarianism, 13
  Vegetarian Society, The,
    223
vitamins, 43, 51, 53, 69, 158,
  186

wafers, 173
  seed wafers, 190

Walker, Norman W, 217 *n* 2
waters, flavoured/sodas, 194,
  213–4
  fizzy water, 214
water retention, 40
wheat/wheat products, 8, 60,
  70
  wheat crisps, 190
whips, 182, 194
wholefoods, 42, 48, 63
  wholefood warehouses, 160
wholegrains, 16
weight loss industry, 74
weight problems, 2, 3, 4, 40,
  75, 113, 140, 166 *see also*
  fat
Wigmore, Ann, 61, 219 *n* 23,
  236
  Ann Wigmore Foundation,
    235
  Ann Wigmore Institute, 235

yoga, 174, 234
yoghurt, 25

Zioudrou, C, 218 *n* 22
zinc, 69